The Finest Anti-Aging Recipes

Reversing the Passage of Time Through Diet

BY Yannick Alcorn

Copyright Warnings

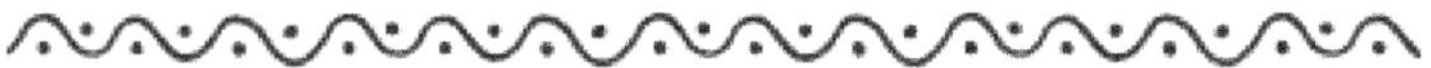

Table of Contents

Introduction

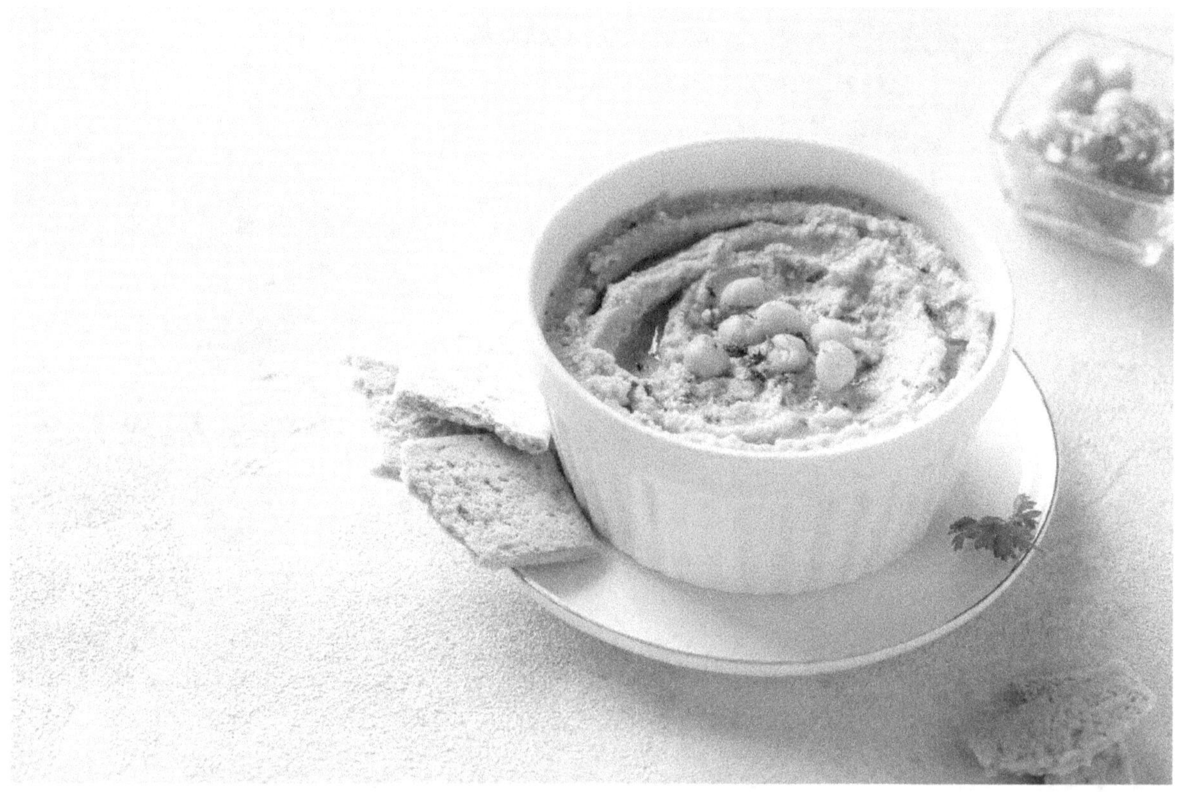

Ensuring a well-rounded diet includes staples; however, there are specific meals that contribute to both feeling and looking fantastic. Each dish in *"The Finest Anti-Aging Dishes,"* comes with a concise explanation of why certain ingredients were chosen, all geared towards promoting youthful qualities. Think of it as a dependable framework that you can modify according to your preferences.

Incorporating not only a wholesome diet but also prioritizing adequate sleep and proper hydration are key factors in preserving youthful radiance. Blend these revitalizing food options with complementary factors in a well-balanced, healthy regimen for enhanced results.

Nurturing both your mental and emotional well-being is made possible through mindful dietary choices and consistent self-care rituals. Make the most of each day on your path to permanent health with the guidance of these recipes.

AAAAAAAAAAAAAAAAAAAAA

1. Crispy Chicken Skin Broccoli Salad

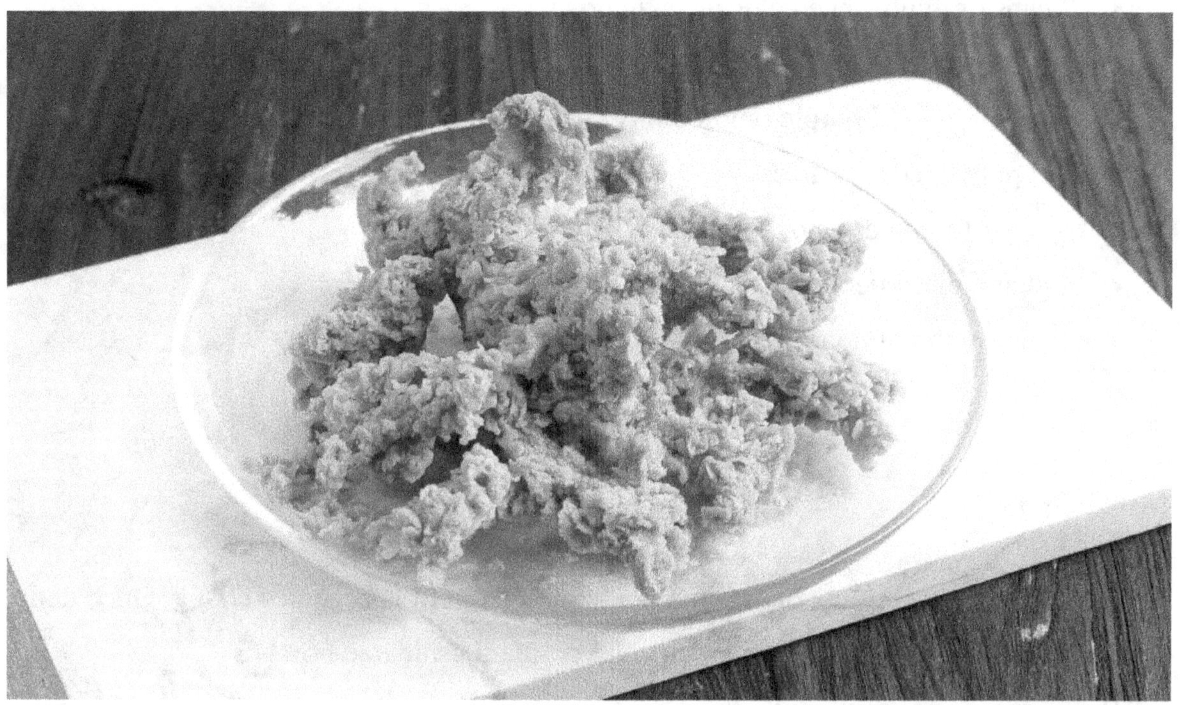

Broccoli is not a favorite vegetable, but if you are looking to boost brain age, this is one vegetable to anti-age your brain.

Duration: 20 minutes

Serving Size: 4

List of Ingredients:

- 2 broccoli florets, chopped including the stalks thinly sliced
- 2 cups of thinly sliced chicken skin crisps
- 4 rations of bacon
- 1 medium-sized purple onion thinly sliced
- 1 cup of shredded carrots
- ½ cup of toasted almond nuts
- Salt and black pepper
- 1 tablespoon of honey

AAAAAAAAAAAAAAAAAAAAA

Instruction:

A. Start by crisping the bacon in a non-stick pan until it becomes crispy. Once done, crumble the bacon into small bits and set them aside in a bowl.

B. In the same bowl with the bacon bits, combine the chopped broccoli florets (including thinly sliced stalks), thinly sliced chicken skin crisps, thinly sliced purple onion, shredded carrots, and toasted almond nuts.

C. To create the dressing, mix honey with the bacon oil left in the pan. Season the dressing with a pinch of salt and black pepper to taste. Drizzle this flavorful dressing over the salad mixture in the bowl.

Cooking Notes:

- When crisping the bacon, you can place the bacon strips in a cold pan and then gradually heat it up. This helps the fat render slowly and results in a crispier texture.
- For the chicken skin crisps, you can make them by removing the skin from chicken pieces, seasoning them with salt and pepper, and then baking them in the oven until they're crispy. Alternatively, you can pan-fry them until crispy.
- When slicing the broccoli stalks thinly, peel off the tough outer layer to reveal the tender part inside before slicing.
- Bacon Selection: Choose high-quality bacon with a good balance of meat and fat for the best results. Thick-cut bacon works well in this recipe, as it crisps up nicely and adds a meaty texture to the salad.
- Chicken Skin Tips: When removing the skin from chicken pieces, try to keep it in larger pieces to make slicing easier. If you're baking the chicken skin, place it on a wire rack to allow air circulation and even cooking.
- Broccoli Texture: To maintain a pleasant texture in the salad, blanch the chopped broccoli florets in boiling water for about 1-2 minutes, then immediately transfer them to an ice water bath to stop the cooking process. This will help the broccoli stay vibrant and slightly crisp.
- Onion Variation: If you prefer a milder onion flavor, you can soak the thinly sliced purple onion in cold water for about 10-15 minutes before adding it to the salad. This helps reduce the sharpness of the onion.
- Carrot Prep: Consider using a vegetable peeler to create thin, long strips of carrots. This adds a delicate crunch and visual appeal to the salad.
- Nut Options: Feel free to experiment with different nuts, such as pine nuts, walnuts, or pecans, for added variety in taste and texture.

- Warm Honey Easily: To warm the honey for the dressing, you can place the honey container in a bowl of warm water for a few minutes or microwave it in short bursts, stirring in between, until it's easier to mix with the bacon oil.
- Serving Ideas: If you want to make this salad more substantial, you can add cooked quinoa, farro, or couscous for extra grains. Grilled shrimp or sliced steak also make great protein additions.
- Storage: If you're making the salad ahead of time, keep the dressing separate until just before serving to maintain the crispiness of the ingredients. Toss the salad just before eating to preserve the textures.
- Customization: Feel free to customize the dressing by adding a splash of apple cider vinegar or Dijon mustard for a tangy kick. Adjust the balance of honey and dressing ingredients to suit your taste preferences.
- Presentation: For an elegant presentation, reserve some toasted almond nuts and bacon bits to sprinkle on top of the salad just before serving, adding an extra layer of crunch and visual appeal.
- Leftovers: Leftover salad can be stored in an airtight container in the refrigerator. Keep in mind that some ingredients, like the bacon and chicken skin, may lose their crispness over time. Re-crisp the chicken skin by briefly reheating it in a hot oven or skillet before adding it to the leftover salad.
- Experiment with Herbs: Adding fresh herbs like chopped parsley, cilantro, or mint can enhance the flavor profile of the salad and provide a burst of freshness.
- Texture Maintenance: If you're concerned about the salad getting soggy when making it ahead of time, consider keeping the toasted almond nuts in a separate container and adding them just before serving to maintain their crunchiness.
- Toast the almond nuts in a dry skillet over medium heat until they turn slightly golden and release a nutty aroma. Keep an eye on them and stir frequently to prevent burning.

- While drizzling the honey over the salad, you can gently warm it to make it easier to mix with the bacon oil. This will help the honey distribute evenly throughout the salad.
- Season the salad with salt and black pepper according to your taste preferences. Start with a small amount and adjust as needed.
- Feel free to adjust the quantities of the ingredients based on your preferences and the number of servings you'd like to make.
- This Crispy Chicken Skin Broccoli Salad can be served as a side dish or a light main course. You can also add grilled chicken or other proteins if desired.
- Before serving, toss the salad well to ensure all the ingredients are coated with the dressing for maximum flavor. Enjoy the combination of crispy textures and savory-sweet flavors in each bite!

2. Colorful Green Olives Mediterranean Salad

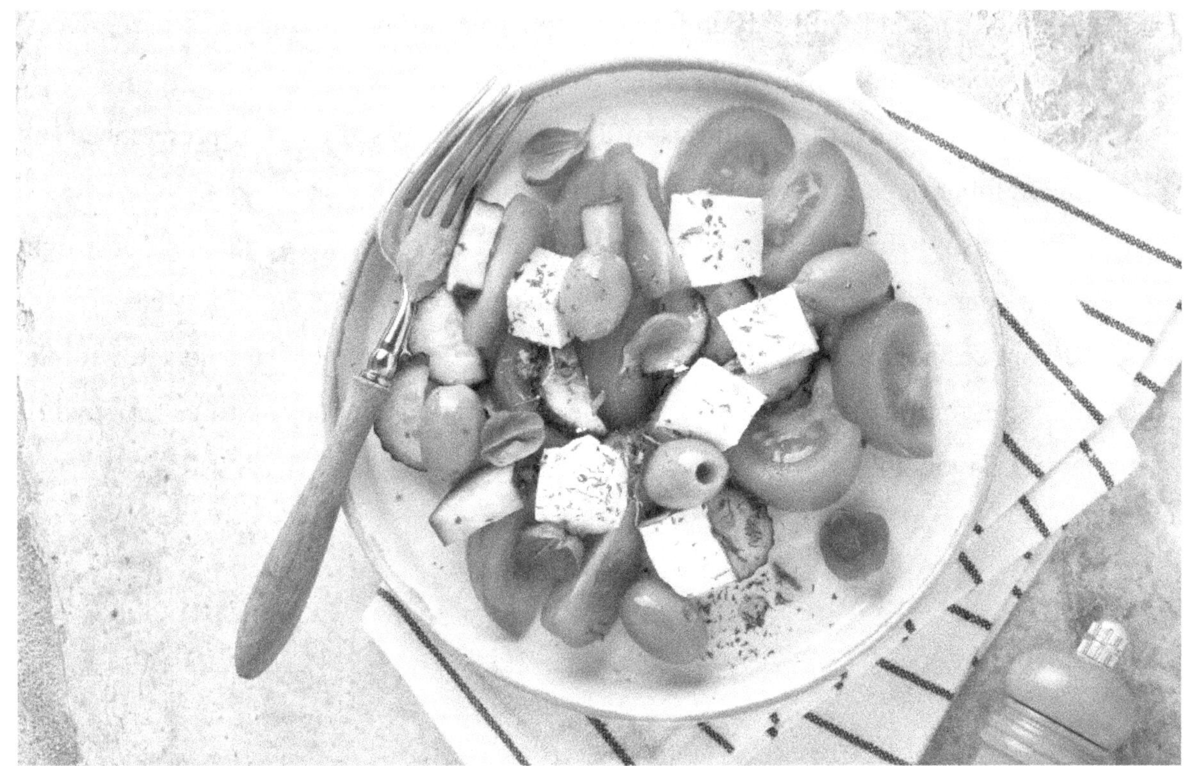

Protect the inside and enjoy a sexy outside with olives. Olives contain polyphenols to keep you youthful and fresh.

Duration: 10 minutes

Serving Size: 4

List of Ingredients:

- 12 colorful tomatoes cut in halves
- 2 dozen fresh green olives, pitted and cut in half
- 1 cup of roughly chopped mint leaves
- A handful of parsley-like a cupful
- Salt and cracked black pepper

Dressing

- 2 tablespoons of olive oil
- 1 teaspoon of garlic, minced
- 2 tablespoons of lemon juice
- 1 teaspoon of Italian dried spices
- Salt and pepper

AAAAAAAAAAAAAAAAAAAAAA

Instruction:

A. Whisk together the dressing ingredients: olive oil, minced garlic, lemon juice, Italian dried spices, salt, and pepper. Set the dressing aside.
B. In a bowl, combine the colorful tomato halves, fresh green olives (pitted and halved), roughly chopped mint leaves, and a handful of chopped parsley.
C. Pour the prepared dressing over the mixture of ingredients in the bowl.
D. Gently toss the salad to ensure that the dressing is evenly distributed and coats all the ingredients.
E. Adjust the seasoning with additional salt and cracked black pepper to taste.
F. Serve the Colorful Green Olives Mediterranean Salad as a refreshing side dish or a light appetizer.

Cooking Notes:

- Choose colorful and ripe tomatoes for the salad to enhance both visual appeal and flavor.
- When cutting the tomatoes, ensure that they are cut into halves to create bite-sized pieces.
- For the fresh green olives, make sure they are pitted and halved to make them easier to eat and enjoy.
- When chopping mint leaves, be gentle to avoid bruising them and releasing too much bitterness.
- Similarly, handle the parsley carefully to maintain its vibrant color and fresh flavor.
- While preparing the dressing, adjust the quantities of garlic, lemon juice, and spices according to your taste preferences.
- Italian dried spices typically include a mix of herbs like basil, oregano, thyme, and rosemary. You can use a pre-made blend or create your own mix.
- When tossing the salad, use a gentle motion to avoid mashing the delicate ingredients.
- Before serving, make sure the salad is well-chilled for a refreshing taste.
- You can customize the salad by adding other Mediterranean-inspired ingredients like feta cheese, red onion slices, or cucumber.
- If you're making the salad ahead of time, consider adding the dressing just before serving to prevent the ingredients from becoming too soggy.
- This salad pairs well with grilled meats, seafood, or can be enjoyed on its own as a light and healthy dish.

3. Beet-Orange Watercress Salad

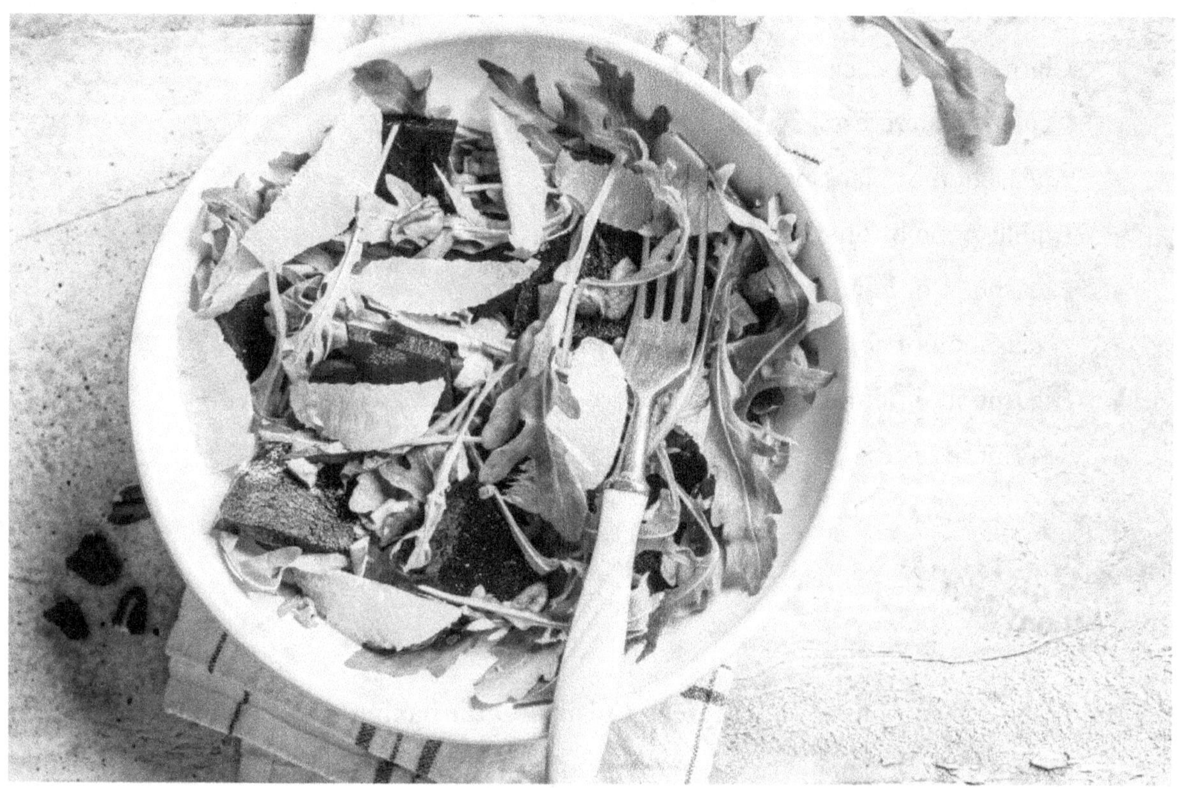

Orange is a vitamin C storehouse, while beets cleanse the liver. A healthy dose of both is a dish for supple and younger-looking skin.

Duration: 90 minutes

Serving Size: 2

List of Ingredients:

- 1 large orange
- 1 large red beet
- 1 large golden beet
- 1 cup of watercress
- ¼ teaspoon of black pepper
- 1 tablespoon of olive oil
- 1 teaspoon of honey
- ¼ teaspoon of chili flakes
- 1 teaspoon of lemon juice
- Sea salt to taste

AAAAAAAAAAAAAAAAAAAAAA

Instruction:

A. Preheat the oven to 205 degrees Celsius. On a baking tray, place the beets and season with salt, pepper, and a drizzle of oil. Roast the beets in the oven until they become soft, which usually takes about 40 to 45 minutes.

B. As the beets approach the end of their roasting time, prepare the orange slices for caramelization. Place the orange slices in the oven to caramelize them slightly.

C. While the beets and oranges are cooking, create the dressing by combining olive oil, honey, lemon juice, and chili flakes. Mix these ingredients together until they are well incorporated.

D. Once the beets are fully roasted and soft, remove them from the oven and allow them to cool down. After cooling, peel the beets and thinly slice them.

E. To assemble the salad, arrange the sliced beets on a plate. Add the watercress on top of the beets to create a bed of greens.

F. Finally, drizzle the prepared dressing over the salad. The combination of flavors from the dressing will enhance the overall taste of the salad.

Cooking Notes:

- When roasting beets, you can wrap them in aluminum foil before placing them on the baking tray. This can help keep moisture in and prevent them from drying out during roasting.
- Caramelizing orange slices adds a sweet and slightly charred flavor to the salad. You can do this by placing the orange slices directly on a baking tray in the oven for a few minutes until they start to caramelize at the edges.
- When preparing the dressing, you can adjust the quantities of honey, lemon juice, and chili flakes to suit your taste preferences. Taste and adjust as needed.
- Make sure the roasted beets are cool enough to handle before peeling and slicing them. You can use gloves to avoid staining your hands with beet juice.
- Watercress adds a peppery and refreshing note to the salad. Wash and dry the watercress leaves before arranging them on the plate.
- To drizzle the dressing evenly, you can use a spoon or a small squeeze bottle. Start with a little dressing and add more if desired.
- Beet Size Consistency: To ensure even roasting, try to select beets of similar size. This will help them cook at a consistent rate and avoid some becoming overcooked while others remain undercooked.
- Orange Zest: Before caramelizing the orange slices, consider grating a bit of orange zest over them for an extra burst of citrus aroma and flavor.
- Chili Flakes Intensity: The heat level of chili flakes can vary, so start with a small amount in the dressing and gradually add more if you prefer a spicier kick. Remember that the heat can intensify as the dressing sits.

- Beet Peeling Tips: After roasting, the beet skins should easily slip off when rubbed gently. If you encounter stubborn areas, a vegetable peeler can help remove any remaining skin.
- Chilling the Beets: For a cooler salad, refrigerate the roasted and sliced beets before assembling the salad. This can be a refreshing option, especially during hot weather.
- Cheese Pairing: Crumbled goat cheese or feta can complement the flavors of the salad. Their creamy texture contrasts nicely with the beets and watercress.
- Nut and Seed Crunch: Consider adding toasted walnuts, pecans, or pumpkin seeds for extra texture and a nutty flavor that pairs well with the other elements of the salad.
- Balsamic Glaze Drizzle: For a tangy and slightly sweet touch, drizzle a balsamic reduction over the salad just before serving. It adds depth and enhances the visual appeal.
- Variation for Vegan Diets: To make this salad vegan, substitute the honey with maple syrup or agave nectar in the dressing, and omit any dairy-based cheese options.
- Herb Garnish: A sprinkle of chopped fresh herbs such as mint, basil, or tarragon can elevate the flavors and add a fragrant element to the salad.
- Temperature Contrast: To balance the warm beets and caramelized orange slices, you can serve the salad on a bed of chilled greens to create an enjoyable temperature contrast.
- Leftovers Transformation: Turn any leftover salad into a grain bowl by adding cooked quinoa, farro, or couscous. The dressing will infuse the grains with delicious flavor.
- Dressing Infusion: Prepare the dressing a bit in advance to allow the flavors to meld. This can enhance the overall taste of the salad.
- Crispy Element: If you're aiming for an additional crunch, consider adding crispy shallots or onions as a garnish on top of the salad.

- Edible Flowers: For a decorative touch, garnish the salad with edible flowers like nasturtiums or pansies. They add visual appeal and a delicate, floral flavor.

- Serve with Crusty Bread: Accompany the salad with a slice of crusty bread or baguette to soak up the flavorful dressing and juices from the beets and oranges.

- Adapt for Seasonal Ingredients: While oranges work well, you can also try using other citrus fruits like grapefruit or blood oranges for a seasonal twist.

- Plate Presentation: Arrange the beets, watercress, and orange slices in an artistic manner, making the dish visually appealing and inviting before drizzling the dressing.

- Refreshing Beverage Pairing: Serve the salad with a refreshing drink like sparkling water with a splash of citrus or a citrus-infused herbal tea to complement the flavors.

- Feel free to add additional elements to the salad, such as goat cheese, nuts, or seeds, to add more texture and flavor.

- This salad can be served as a light appetizer, a side dish, or a refreshing main course. It's particularly enjoyable during warmer months.

- Experiment with the arrangement of beets, watercress, and orange slices to create an appealing presentation.

- Before serving, toss the salad gently to ensure that the dressing coats all the ingredients evenly for a well-balanced taste.

4. Tamarind Flavored Carrot Oatmeal Cookies

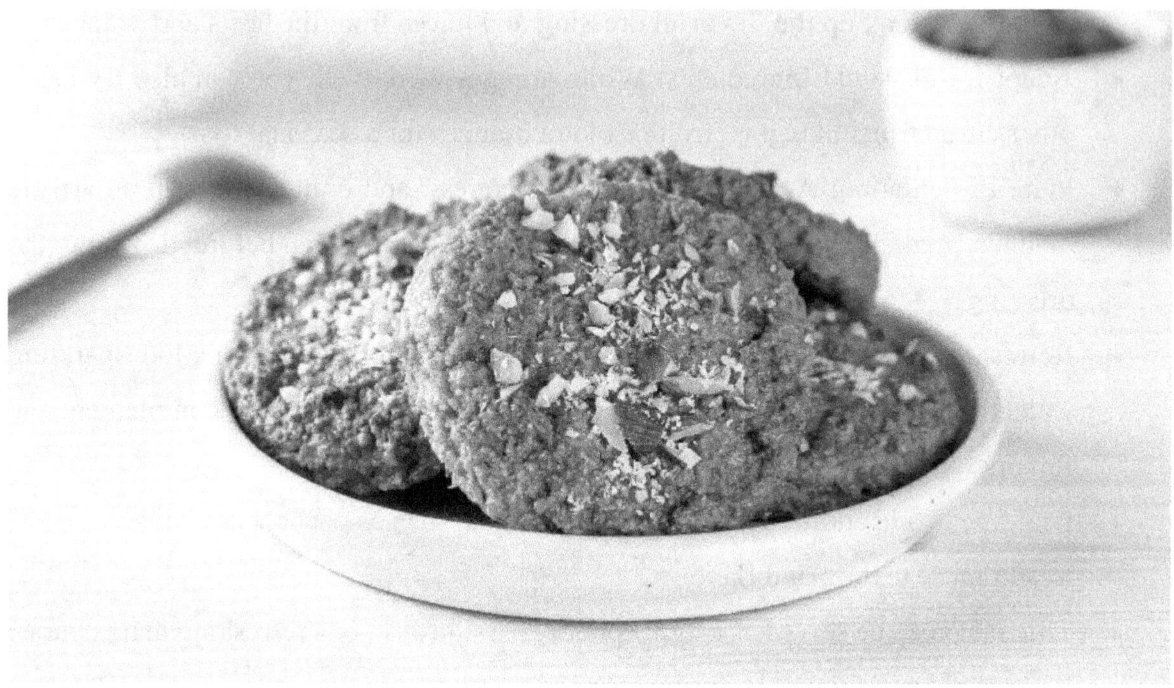

What a healthy combination packed with fiber, flavor, and nutrients.

Baking Temp 325 F

Duration: 35 minutes

Make about 12 cookies

List of Ingredients:

- 1 teaspoon of cinnamon
- ½ teaspoon of nutmeg
- 1 teaspoon of ginger powder
- 2 cups of shredded carrots
- 1 ½ cups of old fashioned oats
- 1 teaspoon of tamarind paste
- 1 tablespoon of brown sugar
- Sea salt
- 1 cup of almond milk

AAAAAAAAAAAAAAAAAAAAAA

Instruction:

A. Use a blender to grind the old-fashioned oats into a flour-like consistency.

B. In a bowl, combine the ground oat flour, cinnamon, nutmeg, ginger powder, shredded carrots, tamarind paste, brown sugar, and a pinch of sea salt.

C. Gradually add almond milk to the mixture in the bowl, stirring until a firm cookie batter is formed.

D. Preheat your oven and line a baking tray with parchment paper.

E. Using a spoon, scoop portions of the cookie batter onto the lined baking tray, forming individual cookies.

F. Bake the cookies in the preheated oven until the edges turn golden brown. This usually takes around 12-15 minutes, but keep an eye on them to avoid over-baking.

G. Once baked, remove the cookies from the oven and allow them to cool on a wire rack.

H. Once the Tamarind Flavored Carrot Oatmeal Cookies have cooled down, they are
ready to be enjoyed.

Cooking Notes:

- Grinding the oats into flour creates a smoother texture for the cookies while still
maintaining the oatmeal's nutritional benefits.
- Tamarind paste adds a unique tangy flavor to the cookies. Adjust the quantity based
on your preference for tanginess.
- Almond milk provides moisture and helps bind the ingredients together. Gradually
adding it ensures the right consistency for the cookie batter.
- Use a lined baking tray to prevent the cookies from sticking and to make the cleanup
process easier.
- The baking time might vary depending on your oven and the size of the cookies.
Keep an eye on them and check for the desired level of browning.
- After removing the cookies from the oven, they will continue to firm up a bit as
they cool. Allow them to cool completely on a wire rack before storing or enjoying.
- Store the cooled cookies in an airtight container to maintain their freshness and
texture.
- Feel free to experiment with the level of sweetness by adjusting the amount of
brown sugar. You can also try using alternative sweeteners like honey or maple
syrup.
- These cookies can be a great treat for a snack or dessert, and the combination of
flavors offers a unique twist on traditional oatmeal cookies.
- If you'd like to add extra crunch and flavor, consider incorporating chopped nuts,
dried fruits, or even shredded coconut to the cookie batter.

- Always be cautious when introducing new ingredients into your diet or your pet's diet. If you're making these cookies for your dog, make sure all the ingredients are safe and suitable for their consumption.

5. Golden Coconut Cookies

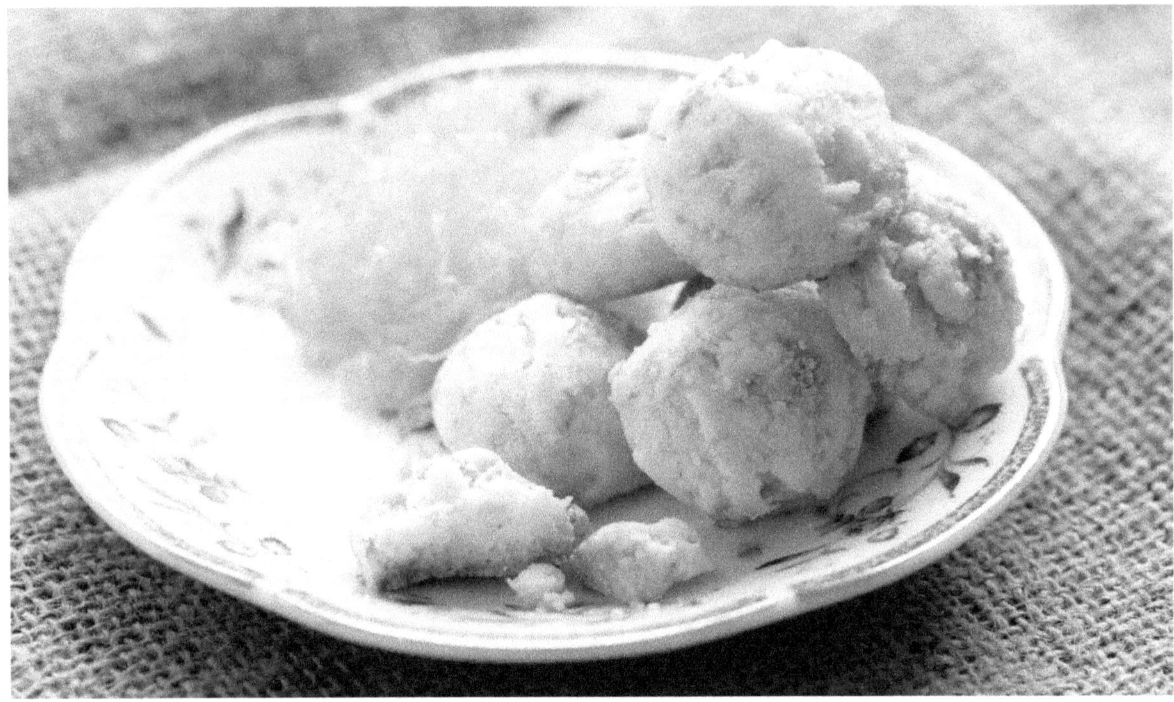

Turmeric is the mother of all spices. Not only does it brighten the food, but it fights damaged cells, and aging and prevents DNA shortening.

Duration: 15 minutes

Serving Size: 16 cookies

List of Ingredients:

- 1 cup of almond flour
- 1 cup of rolled oat
- ½ cup of sweetened coconut flakes
- 1 teaspoon of ground turmeric
- 1 teaspoon of ginger powder
- ½ teaspoon of baking powder
- ½ teaspoon of nutmeg
- ½ cup of hydrated raisins
- ¼ teaspoon of sea salt
- 40 ml of clarified butter
- 1 teaspoon of coconut extract
- 3 tablespoons of honey

AAAAAAAAAAAAAAAAAAAAAA

Instruction:

A. Start by adding all the dry ingredients to a bowl. This includes coconut flour, almond flour, baking powder, and a pinch of salt.

B. Pour in the clarified butter (ghee), honey, and vanilla extract into the bowl with the dry ingredients.

C. Mix the ingredients together until they form a cohesive dough. Apply some pressure while mixing to ensure everything combines well.

D. Use a spoon or scoop to form balls from the dough. Place the dough balls on a baking tray lined with parchment paper.

E. Preheat your oven and then place the tray with the dough balls into the oven. Bake the cookies at the specified temperature for around 12 minutes.

F. Keep an eye on the cookies and remove them from the oven once they have turned golden brown.

G. Allow the cookies to cool completely before sharing or storing them.

Cooking Notes:

- Coconut flour and almond flour give these cookies a unique texture and flavor. Make sure to use finely ground flours for best results.

- Clarified butter (ghee) adds richness to the cookies. It's a common ingredient in many Indian recipes and offers a wonderful aroma.

- Honey provides natural sweetness to the cookies. Adjust the amount according to your taste preference.

- Vanilla extract enhances the overall flavor profile of the cookies. You can also experiment with other extracts like almond or coconut.

- Mixing the dough well ensures that all the dry and wet ingredients are evenly distributed for consistent taste and texture.

- When forming dough balls, you can make them as big or small as you like, depending on your preference.

- Baking time may vary slightly based on your oven, so keep an eye on the cookies to avoid over-baking.

- Allow the cookies to cool on a wire rack after removing them from the oven. This helps them become crispier as they cool.

- The texture of coconut flour can vary, so the dough might feel a bit crumbly. Applying pressure while mixing and shaping the cookies will help them hold together.

- These Golden Coconut Cookies are suitable for sharing as a healthy treat or snack. They're also great for those following gluten-free or paleo diets.

- Store the cooled cookies in an airtight container to maintain their freshness and texture.

- Flour Consistency: Make sure your coconut flour and almond flour are well sifted and free of any lumps. This will ensure a smooth and consistent texture in the cookies.

- Room Temperature Ingredients: Using room temperature clarified butter (ghee), honey, and eggs can make mixing and incorporating the ingredients easier and more efficient.

- Adding Optional Mix-Ins: Consider adding mix-ins like chocolate chips, chopped nuts, dried fruits, or shredded coconut to add extra flavor, texture, and variety to the cookies.

- Chilling the Dough: If the dough seems too soft or sticky to handle, you can chill it in the refrigerator for about 15-30 minutes before shaping it into balls. This can make the dough easier to work with.

- Uniform Size: Use a cookie scoop to portion out the dough for consistent cookie size. This helps ensure even baking and a uniform appearance.

- Flattening the Dough Balls: Gently flatten the dough balls slightly with the palm of your hand or the back of a spoon before baking. This can help the cookies spread and bake evenly.

- Monitor Baking Time: Baking times can vary based on the size of the cookies and individual ovens. Check the cookies around the 10-minute mark to prevent them from becoming too dark.

- Cooling Rack Benefits: Cooling the cookies on a wire rack rather than on the baking tray allows air to circulate around the cookies, preventing them from becoming soggy on the bottom.

- Flavor Variations: Experiment with adding spices like cinnamon, nutmeg, or cardamom to the dough for extra warmth and depth of flavor.

- Sweetener Alternatives: If you prefer a different sweetener, you can use maple syrup, agave nectar, or a sugar substitute suitable for baking. Adjust the quantities based on the sweetness level you desire.

- Storing with Freshness: To maintain the cookies' crispy texture, you can add a piece of bread to the container with the cookies. The bread will help absorb excess moisture and keep the cookies crisp.

- Nut-Free Option: If nut allergies are a concern, consider using seed flours like sunflower seed flour or pumpkin seed flour as an alternative to almond flour.

- Freezing Cookies: These cookies freeze well. Place them in an airtight container with layers of parchment paper between each layer to prevent sticking. Thaw at room temperature before enjoying.

- Healthy Fat Source: Clarified butter (ghee) provides a healthy source of fat for these cookies. It has a higher smoke point than regular butter, making it suitable for baking at higher temperatures.

- Balancing Sweetness: If you find the cookies too sweet, you can reduce the amount of honey while still maintaining the desired consistency of the dough.

- Presentation Ideas: Dust the cooled cookies with a light sprinkle of powdered sugar or drizzle with a simple glaze made from powdered sugar and a touch of milk or lemon juice for an elegant touch.

- Texture Exploration: These cookies have a delicate crumb due to the flours used. If you prefer a chewier texture, you can experiment with adding a small amount of tapioca flour or arrowroot starch to the mixture.

- Family-Friendly Activity: These cookies are a great baking project to involve kids in the kitchen. They can help mix the dough and shape the cookies, making it a fun and educational experience.

- Always be cautious when introducing new ingredients into your diet or someone else's, especially if there are allergies or sensitivities to consider.

6. Spicy Ghee Roasted Plantains

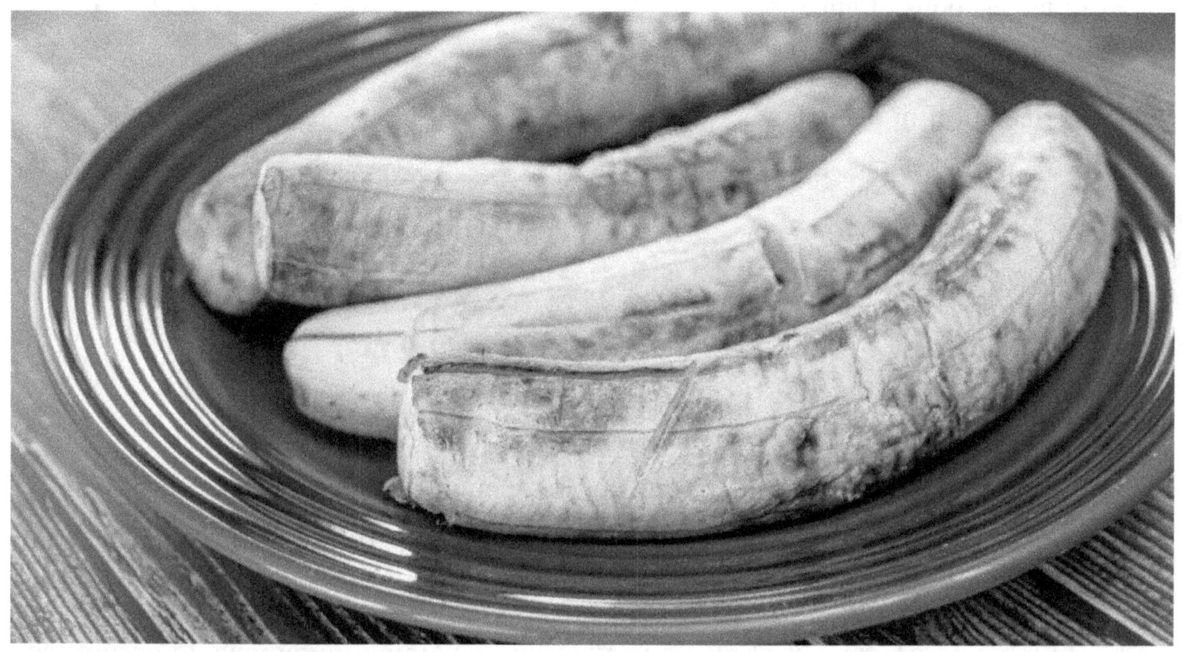

Ghee is a healthy fat that reduces cholesterol while plantains are tasty, full of fiber, improve your mood, and solve constipation.

Duration: 325 F

Cooking time 25 minutes

Serving Size: 4

List of Ingredients:

- 1 teaspoon of garlic
- 2 tablespoons of ghee
- A dash of chili flakes
- 3 ripe but firm plantains
- 1 tablespoon of coconut sugar (optional)
- A sprinkle of sea salt

AAAAAAAAAAAAAAAAAAAA

Instruction:

A. Begin by peeling the plantains and cutting them diagonally into slices.

B. Preheat the oven, allowing it to heat for about 5 to 10 minutes before you start roasting the plantains.

C. In a bowl, toss the sliced plantains with the remaining ingredients to ensure they are well coated.

D. Arrange the coated plantain slices in a single layer on a parchment paper-lined baking sheet.

E. Place the baking sheet with the plantains in the preheated oven and roast them until the underside becomes browned and caramelized.

F. Once the underside is browned, flip the plantain slices to the other side to ensure even roasting.

G. After both sides are nicely roasted and the plantains are tender, remove them from the oven.

H. Serve the Spicy Ghee Roasted Plantains with a sprinkle of sea salt for added flavor.

Cooking Notes:

- Cutting the plantains diagonally creates larger slices that are easier to handle and have more surface area for roasting.
- Preheating the oven before roasting helps ensure that the plantains start cooking immediately once they're placed inside.
- Tossing the plantains in the bowl with the spices and ghee ensures even coating for better flavor distribution.
- Placing the coated plantains on parchment paper prevents sticking and makes cleanup easier.
- Roasting the plantains at a high temperature helps caramelize the natural sugars in the fruit, creating a delicious caramelized exterior.
- When flipping the plantain slices, use tongs or a spatula to avoid burning your fingers.
- Sea salt adds a final touch to enhance the flavors. You can adjust the amount of salt to your taste preference.
- These Spicy Ghee Roasted Plantains can be served as a side dish, snack, or even as a unique addition to a salad or main course.
- Customize the level of spiciness by adjusting the quantity of spices used. You can also experiment with different spice blends.
- Ensure that the plantains are ripe but not overly ripe for the best texture and flavor.
- Ghee, a form of clarified butter, imparts a rich flavor and aids in browning during roasting.
- Serve the roasted plantains warm for the best taste and texture experience.
- Experiment with additional toppings or sauces like yogurt, lime juice, or a drizzle of honey for extra flavor variations.
- Always be cautious when handling hot trays or utensils from the oven. Use oven mitts or gloves to prevent burns.

- Enjoy the combination of sweet, spicy, and savory flavors in each bite of these Spicy Ghee Roasted Plantains!

7. Creamy Cheesy Nutty Grapes Salad

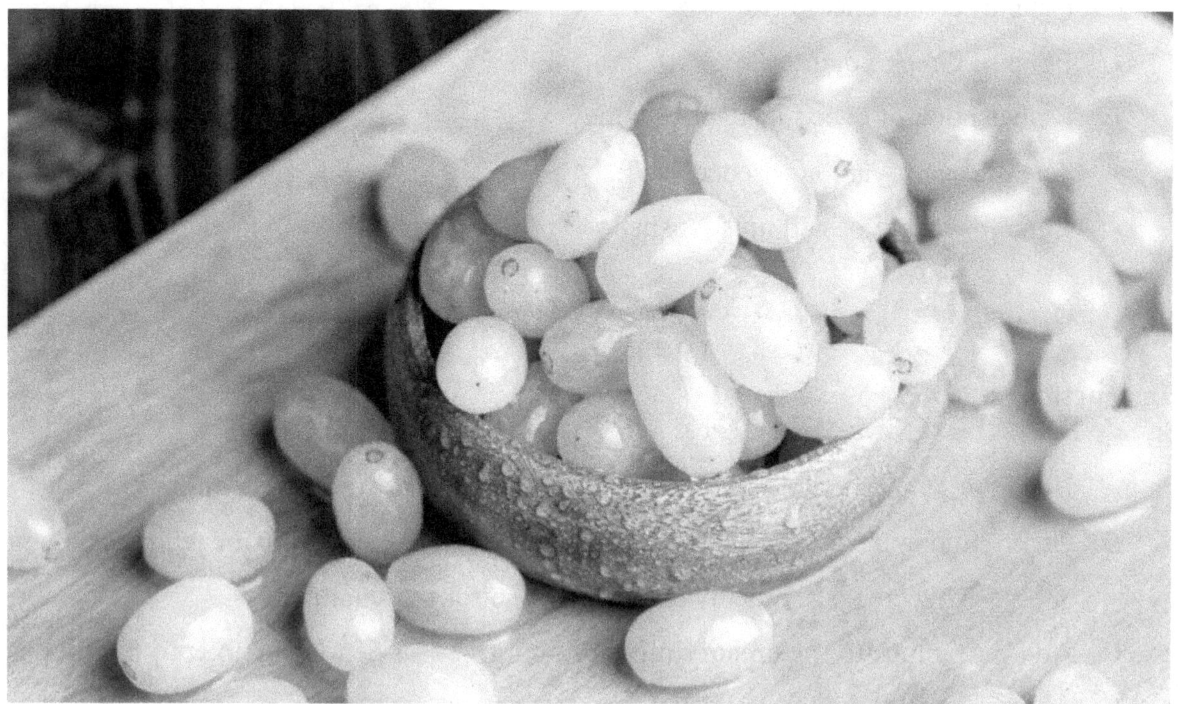

This skin-healing combination is great for breakfast, lunch, or dinner and is packed with proteins and antioxidants.

Duration: 12 minutes

Serving Size: 4

List of Ingredients:

- 4 cups of red and green grapes
- 1 cup of cream cheese
- 1 cup of Greek yogurt
- 1 tablespoon of coconut sugar or honey
- ½ teaspoon of vanilla essence
- 1 cup of mixed toasted nuts crushed

AAAAAAAAAAAAAAAAAAAAA

Instruction:

A. Begin by whipping the cream cheese until it becomes fluffy in texture.
B. Gently fold in the coconut sugar, yogurt, and vanilla extract into the whipped cream cheese. This creates a creamy and sweet base for the salad.
C. Add the grapes to the creamy mixture and give it a gentle stir to coat the grapes evenly with the creamy and cheesy mixture.
D. Once the grapes are well-coated, refrigerate the mixture to chill and allow the flavors to meld.
E. Before serving, sprinkle the nuts over the creamy grape mixture. The nuts add a delightful crunch and nutty flavor to the salad.

Cooking Notes:

- Use softened cream cheese for easy whipping and smoother incorporation into the salad.
- Coconut sugar provides a natural sweetness and complements the flavors of the grapes and creamy components.

- Yogurt adds tanginess and additional creaminess to the mixture. Opt for plain yogurt without added sugars or flavors.
- Vanilla extract enhances the overall flavor profile of the creamy mixture. You can also experiment with other flavor extracts if desired.
- Use a variety of grapes for a colorful and flavorful salad. Red, green, or black grapes all work well.
- Stirring the grapes gently ensures that they are coated with the creamy mixture without getting crushed.
- Refrigerating the salad before serving allows the flavors to develop and the creamy mixture to set slightly.
- Nuts provide texture and a contrasting element to the creamy and juicy grapes. Chopped walnuts, almonds, or pecans can work well.
- You can serve this Creamy Cheesy Nutty Grapes Salad as a side dish, dessert, or a light and refreshing snack.
- Cream Cheese Temperature: Allow the cream cheese to come to room temperature before whipping. Softened cream cheese blends more smoothly and prevents lumps in the creamy mixture.
- Even Coconut Sugar Distribution: To ensure the coconut sugar mixes evenly, you can sift it before folding it into the whipped cream cheese. This prevents any clumps from forming.
- Yogurt Variation: Greek yogurt can be a great option as it offers creaminess and a slightly tangy flavor. Adjust the amount of yogurt based on your desired level of tanginess.
- Chill the Mixing Bowl: For better whipping results, you can chill the mixing bowl and beaters in the refrigerator for about 15 minutes before whipping the cream cheese.
- Grapes Prep: Wash and pat dry the grapes before adding them to the creamy mixture. Removing excess moisture helps the creamy coating adhere better.

- Serving Size Consideration: The size of the grape clusters can vary, so adjust the number of clusters used based on your desired serving size.

- Chill Time Optimization: While chilling the salad for at least an hour is recommended for optimal flavor melding, you can also serve it immediately if you're short on time. The flavors will continue to develop as it chills.

- Nuts as a Garnish: You can toast the nuts lightly before adding them to the salad. This enhances their flavor and adds a nice aroma to the dish.

- Honey Drizzle: For a touch of extra sweetness, consider drizzling a small amount of honey over the salad just before serving.

- Fresh Fruit Addition: To add more variety to the salad, you can include other bite-sized fruits like berries or diced melon. These can enhance the colors and flavors.

- Cream Cheese Alternatives: If you're looking for a dairy-free option, you can use a vegan cream cheese or a blended silken tofu for the creamy base.

- Storage Tips: If you have leftovers, store the salad in an airtight container in the refrigerator. Gently toss the salad before serving again to redistribute the creamy mixture.

- Garnish Options: Along with nuts, you can garnish the salad with shredded coconut, grated dark chocolate, or a sprinkle of cinnamon for added visual appeal.

- Use Ripe Grapes: Choose ripe and plump grapes for the best flavor. Avoid overly mushy or under ripe grapes.

- Layered Presentation: For an elegant touch, layer the creamy mixture and grapes in individual serving glasses or bowls, alternating between the two.

- Pairing with Wine: This salad can be a delightful accompaniment to a glass of white wine, such as a slightly sweet Riesling or a sparkling Moscato.

- Dietary Adjustments: To make the salad lower in sugar, you can reduce the amount of coconut sugar or use a sugar substitute like stevia.

- Gentle Mixing: When folding in the ingredients, use a light hand to avoid overmixing and maintain the integrity of the grapes.

- Balanced Flavors: Taste the creamy mixture before chilling and adjust the sweetness or tanginess by adding more coconut sugar or yogurt, respectively.

- Preparation Ahead: You can prepare the creamy mixture in advance and keep it chilled until ready to serve. Add the grapes and nuts just before serving for optimal freshness.

- Make sure the salad is well-chilled before serving, especially if you're serving it on a warm day.

- Experiment with different nuts or seeds to suit your taste preferences and any potential allergies.

- Feel free to add other complementary ingredients such as fresh mint leaves for an added burst of freshness.

- This salad is best enjoyed on the day it's prepared to maintain the optimal texture and flavor of the grapes.

- Serve the salad in individual bowls or as part of a buffet-style spread.

- Consider the dietary restrictions and preferences of your guests when making this dish, especially if there are allergies or sensitivities to certain ingredients.

8. Pomegranate Dark Chocolate Barks

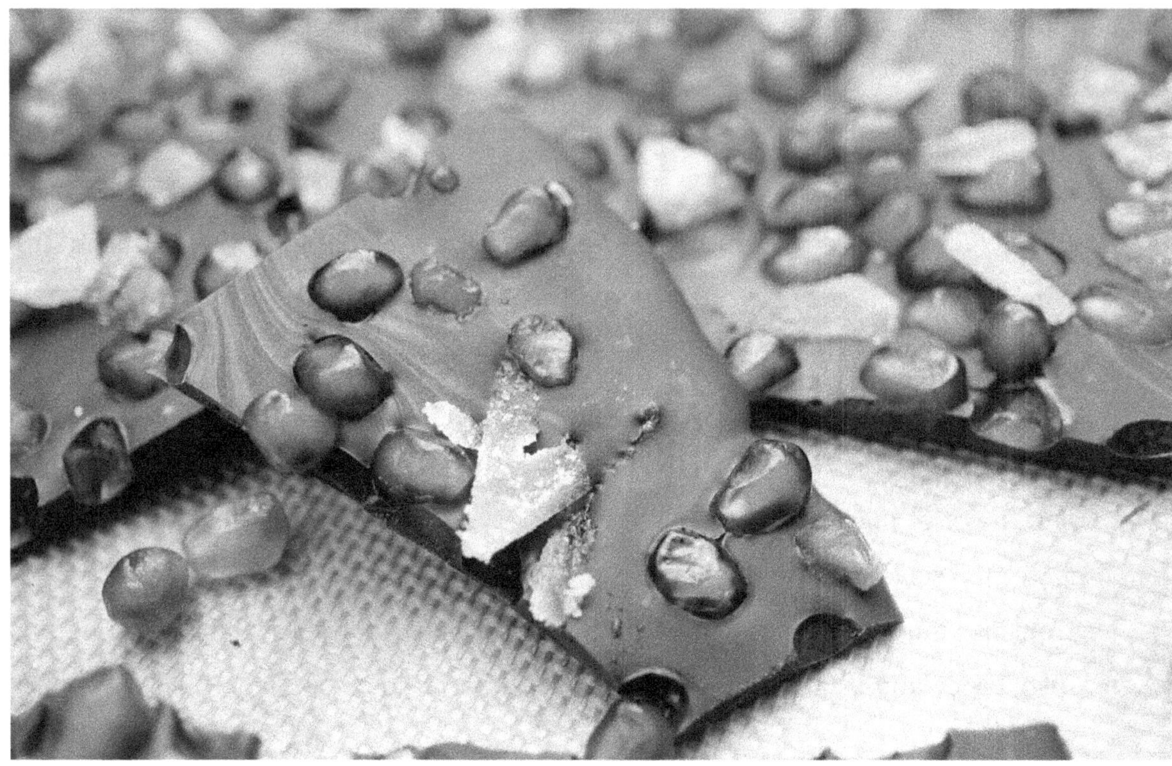

Pomegranate contains chemicals that help your body fight free radicals and preserve Size: collagen for healthier skin.

Duration: 15 minutes

Serving Size: 16 barks

List of Ingredients:

- ½ cup of pomegranate arils
- 400g of dark chocolate chips
- ¼ cup of smoked coconut bark
- 2 tablespoons of crystalline ginger bits
- A sprinkle of sea salt as desired

AAAAAAAAAAAAAAAAAAAAAA

Instruction:

A. Begin by melting the dark chocolate using a double boiler method, which involves placing a heatproof bowl over a pot of simmering water.

B. Once the chocolate is fully melted, continue stirring it even after removing it from the heat source. Monitor the temperature and aim for it to cool down to around 27 degrees Celsius.

C. Return the chocolate to the double boiler, still stirring, until it reaches a temperature of about 32 degrees Celsius. At this stage, the chocolate should have a shiny, smooth, and glossy appearance.

D. After achieving the desired texture and temperature, carefully pour the melted chocolate onto a flat tray lined with parchment paper.

E. Sprinkle the pomegranate seeds over the melted chocolate, ensuring an even distribution.

F. Allow the chocolate bark to set. You can do this at room temperature or, if you're in a hurry, place the tray in the refrigerator for faster setting.

G. Once the chocolate has completely set and hardened, break it into pieces by hand or using a knife.

H. Indulge your sweet tooth by enjoying the Pomegranate Dark Chocolate Barks as a delicious treat.

Cooking Notes:

- Dark chocolate with a high cocoa content works best for making chocolate barks.
- Using a double boiler prevents the chocolate from direct contact with high heat, which can cause it to burn or seize.
- Stirring the chocolate during the cooling process helps in achieving a smooth and well-tempered texture.
- Temperature control is crucial in tempering chocolate properly. The process of raising and lowering the chocolate's temperature helps give it the desired shine and snap.
- Pomegranate seeds add a burst of sweetness and a delightful crunch to the chocolate bark.
- Ensure that the parchment paper on the flat tray is larger than the tray itself, so it's easier to remove the bark once it's set.
- Letting the chocolate bark set allows it to harden and maintain its shape when broken into pieces.
- If you're in a hurry, placing the tray in the refrigerator can speed up the setting process.
- Store the chocolate bark in an airtight container in a cool, dry place to prevent it from melting or becoming too soft.
- This Pomegranate Dark Chocolate Bark can be a wonderful homemade gift or a delectable dessert to enjoy on special occasions.
- Customize the recipe by adding other toppings like chopped nuts, dried fruits, or even a sprinkle of sea salt for a sweet-savory combination.

- Always be cautious when handling hot materials or sharp tools in the kitchen. Use oven mitts or gloves and handle knives carefully.

- Be mindful of portion sizes when enjoying chocolate treats, as they can be calorie-dense.

- Consider dietary preferences and allergies when sharing or gifting chocolate barks.

9. Collagen Baked Sweet Potato Waffle

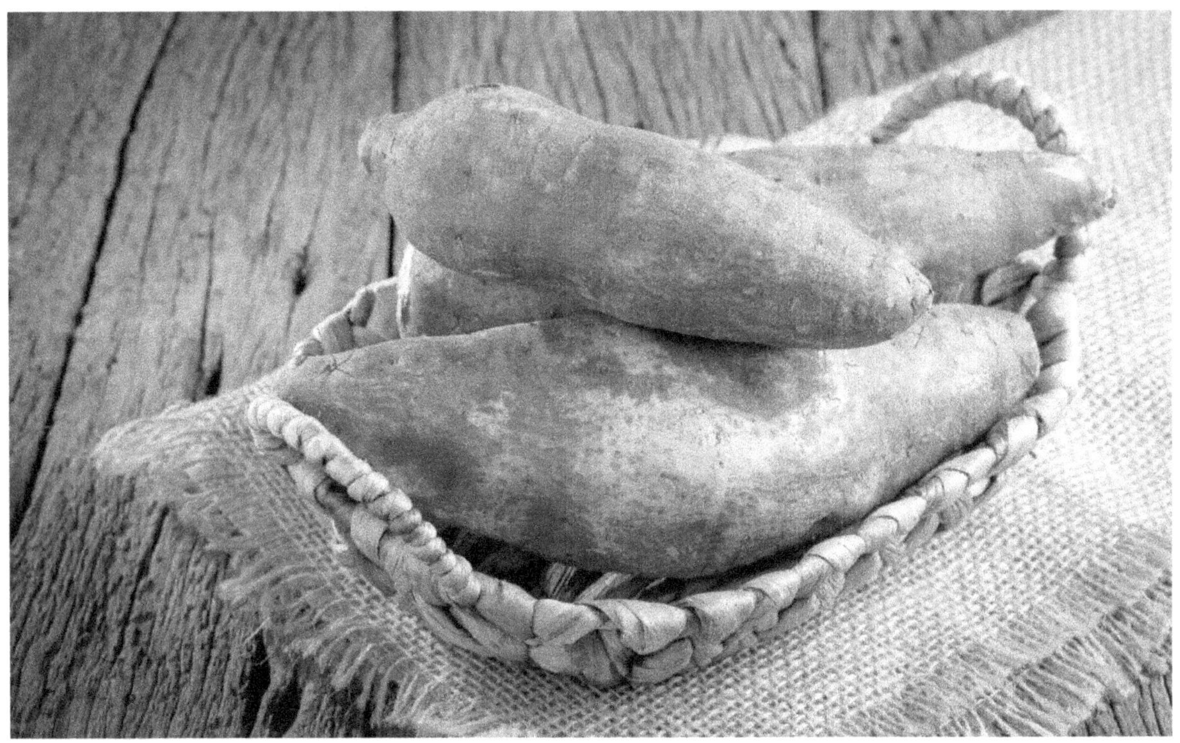

Wrinkles and fine lines an issue boost your collagen supply with this healthy and delicious sweet potato recipe.

Duration: 15 minutes

Serving Size: 2

List of Ingredients:

- 1 cup of mashed sweet potatoes
- 1 egg white
- 1 whole egg
- 1 cup of coconut flour
- ½ cup of milk
- ½ teaspoon of baking powder
- Salt
- 1 tablespoon of coconut oil

AAAAAAAAAAAAAAAAAAAAAA

Instruction:

A. Begin by whipping together the mashed sweet potatoes, egg white, whole egg, coconut flour, milk, baking powder, a pinch of salt, and coconut oil in a bowl. Set this batter aside while you preheat the waffle iron.

B. Once the waffle iron is heated, lightly spray the surface with cooking oil to prevent sticking.

C. Pour the prepared batter onto the waffle iron's surface. Close the waffle iron's lid and allow the batter to cook and set according to the waffle iron's instructions.

D. Repeat the process of pouring the batter and cooking until all the batter is used and you have made the desired number of waffles.

E. Once the Collagen Baked Sweet Potato Waffles are cooked and have a golden-brown color, remove them from the waffle iron.

F. For serving, you have the option to enjoy the waffles with a variety of toppings. For breakfast, consider adding any fruit of your choice along with Greek yogurt. For lunch, you can pair the waffles with chili or other savory toppings.

Cooking Notes:

- Mashed sweet potatoes add natural sweetness, flavor, and moisture to the waffle batter.
- Using both egg white and whole egg helps in binding the ingredients and providing structure to the waffles.
- Coconut flour is a gluten-free flour that contributes to the texture of the waffles.
- Baking powder helps the waffles rise and become fluffy.
- Coconut oil is used to prevent sticking and adds a subtle coconut flavor.
- Preheating the waffle iron ensures that the batter cooks evenly and forms a crispy exterior.
- Lightly spraying the waffle iron's surface with oil prevents the waffles from sticking and makes them easier to remove.
- Cooking times may vary based on the waffle iron's size and specifications. Follow the manufacturer's instructions for best results.
- Toppings can be personalized to your preference. Fresh fruits and Greek yogurt add a healthy and delicious touch to breakfast, while savory options like chili make the waffles suitable for lunch or dinner.
- Consistency of Mashed Sweet Potatoes: Ensure that the mashed sweet potatoes are smooth and free of lumps to create a uniform texture in the waffle batter.
- Batter Resting Time: Allowing the batter to rest for a few minutes before cooking can help the coconut flour absorb the liquids and thicken the batter slightly.
- Milk Choices: You can use any milk of your choice – dairy or non-dairy – based on your dietary preferences. Unsweetened almond milk, coconut milk, or regular milk all work well.
- Alternative Flours: If you want to experiment with the recipe, you can try using other gluten-free flours such as almond flour or oat flour in place of coconut flour. Keep in mind that the texture and flavor may vary.

- Toppings Variety: Get creative with toppings! Consider adding nut butters, chia seeds, honey, maple syrup, or a dusting of cocoa powder for extra flavor and nutrition.

- Waffle Iron Types: Different waffle irons have different heating elements and sizes. Adjust the amount of batter poured accordingly to avoid overflow or underfilling.

- Temperature Adjustment: If your waffle iron has adjustable temperature settings, you can experiment with different levels of browning to achieve your preferred level of crispiness.

- Flavor Enhancements: Add a pinch of cinnamon, nutmeg, or vanilla extract to the batter for additional warmth and flavor complexity.

- Meal Prep: You can make a larger batch of waffles and freeze them individually for a quick breakfast option. Reheat them in the toaster or oven straight from the freezer.

- Serving Suggestions: Along with sweet and savory toppings, consider serving these waffles with a side salad or steamed vegetables for a balanced meal.

- Texture Adjustments: If you prefer a lighter texture, separate the egg yolks from the whites. Beat the egg whites until stiff peaks form and fold them into the batter just before cooking for extra fluffiness.

- Vegan Adaptation: To make these waffles vegan, you can replace the eggs with flax or chia seed eggs, and use plant-based milk and oil.

- Waffle Shape and Size: Play around with waffle iron shapes – round, square, or even fun shapes for a playful twist, especially if serving to children.

- Collagen Powder Consideration: If you're using collagen powder, opt for a flavorless and odorless variety to prevent altering the taste of the waffles.

- Texture Testing: The first waffle might be a bit of a test, so adjust batter consistency or cooking time if needed for subsequent batches.

- Leftover Waffle Ideas: Transform leftover waffles into sandwiches with fillings like scrambled eggs, avocado, and cheese, or use them as a base for mini pizzas.

- Storage and Reheating: Store leftover waffles in a zip-top bag or airtight container in the freezer. To reheat, use a toaster or oven at a low temperature until warmed through.

- Customization: These waffles are versatile – feel free to modify the recipe by incorporating protein powder, adding grated vegetables, or using different spices to suit your taste and nutritional needs.

- Collagen is known for its potential health benefits, including supporting joint and skin health. Make sure to use a high-quality collagen powder if you choose to add it to your waffle batter.

- These Collagen Baked Sweet Potato Waffles can be a creative and nutritious addition to your meal routine, offering a balance of carbohydrates, protein, and healthy fats.

- Store any leftover waffles in an airtight container and reheat them in a toaster or oven for a quick and convenient meal.

- Experiment with different toppings, spices, and mix-ins to create your own unique waffle variations.

- Always adjust portion sizes and ingredients according to your dietary needs and preferences.

10. Spinach Stewed Green Lentil

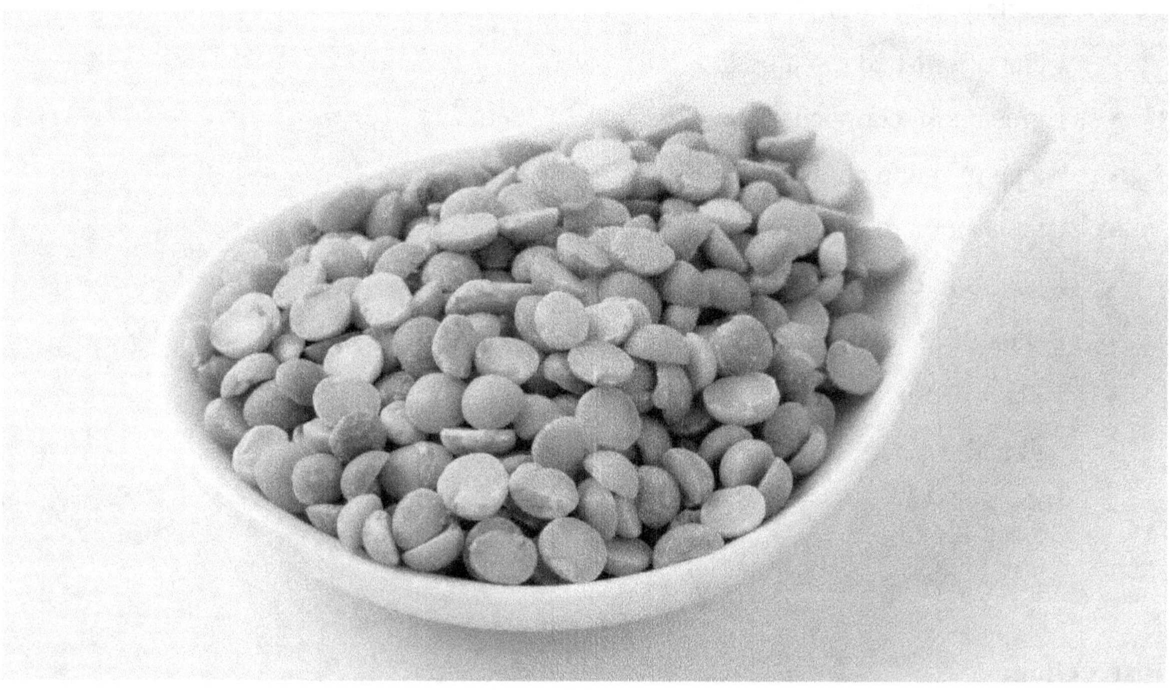

Lentil is a legume with lots of benefits and combining it with spinach takes these superfoods up a notch.

Duration: 55 minutes

Serving Size: 4

List of Ingredients:

- 2 cups of green lentils
- 2 tablespoons of olive oil
- 1 cup of crushed tomatoes
- 1 green chili chopped
- ½ cup of onion chopped
- 1 tablespoon of tomato paste
- 1 teaspoon of minced garlic
- 1 stalk of leek chopped
- 500g of fresh spinach
- Salt and pepper
- 1000 ml of water or chicken stock

AAAAAAAAAAAAAAAAAAAAA

Instruction:

A. Begin by using a slow cooker. Add oil to the slow cooker and sauté the onion, garlic, and leeks until they become softened.

B. After sautéing the aromatics, add the crushed tomatoes and tomato paste to the slow cooker. Cook the mixture for about a minute, and then add the green lentils.

C. Pour in the stock to the slow cooker and cover it with the lid. Allow the lentil mixture to cook.

D. After approximately 30 minutes, check the lentils to see if they have softened. If they have, it's time to add the spinach to the mixture.

E. Once the spinach is added, season the stew well with your preferred seasonings.

F. The Spinach Stewed Green Lentil is now ready to be served and enjoyed.

Cooking Notes:

- Sautéing the onion, garlic, and leeks in oil helps develop the base flavors of the stew.
- Adding crushed tomatoes and tomato paste provides a rich tomato flavor to the dish.
- Green lentils are a good choice for stews, as they hold their shape well and provide a slightly nutty taste.
- Adding stock to the slow cooker provides the necessary liquid for cooking the lentils and creating a flavorful broth.
- Cooking times may vary depending on your slow cooker's settings and the type of lentils used. The goal is to have tender lentils without them becoming mushy.
- Adding spinach towards the end of cooking prevents it from overcooking and maintains its vibrant color and nutrients.
- Season the stew according to your taste preferences. You can use herbs, spices, and salt to enhance the flavors.
- Serve the Spinach Stewed Green Lentil as a hearty and nutritious meal on its own or pair it with bread, rice, or a side salad.
- Leftovers can be stored in an airtight container in the refrigerator. Reheat gently on the stove or in the microwave.
- Experiment with adding other vegetables, such as carrots, bell peppers, or celery, to enhance the nutritional value and flavor profile of the stew.
- Slow cookers offer convenience and allow for a hands-off cooking approach. They're great for making hearty and flavorful dishes like this stew.
- Adjust the seasonings and ingredients based on your dietary preferences and needs.
- This Spinach Stewed Green Lentil recipe can be customized to suit various dietary requirements, including vegetarian and vegan diets.

11. Coconut Coated Oven Baked Tomato Chips

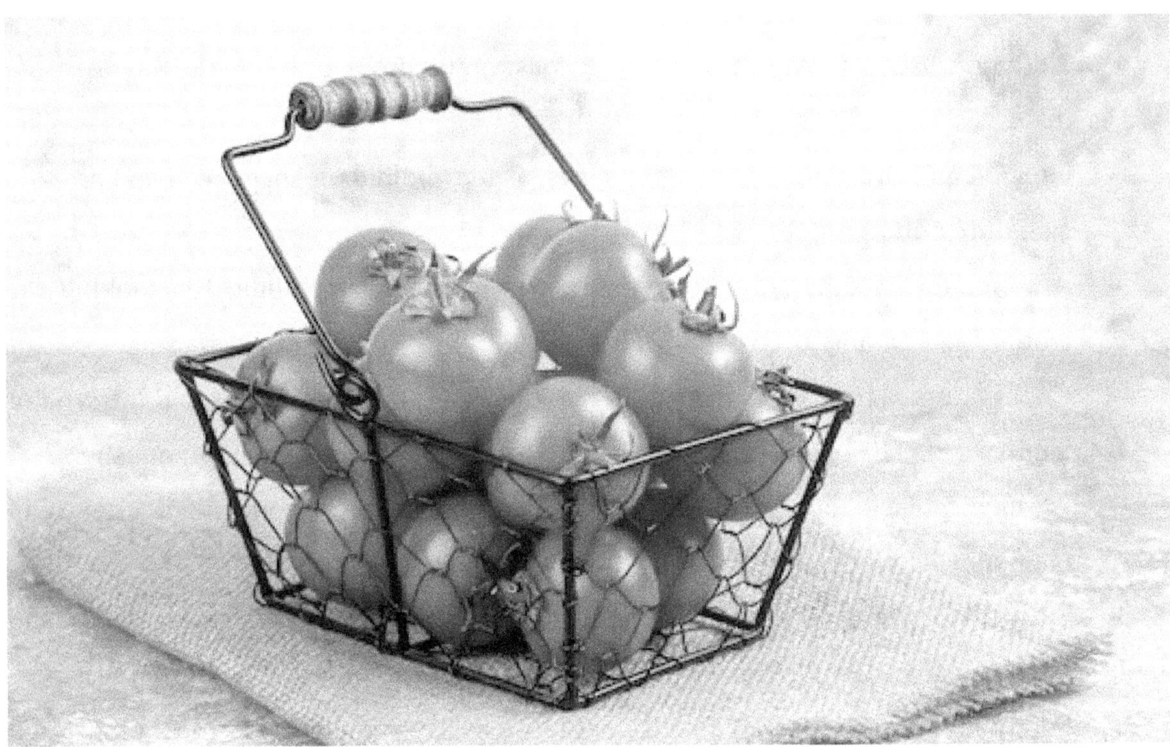

Tomatoes are the number one ingredient containing a component that protects your skin from damage –lycopene. This simple trick will have you eating tomatoes instead of packed potato chips.

Duration: 6-8 hours

Serving Size: 1

List of Ingredients:

- 4 plum tomatoes sliced ½ inch thick
- 2 tablespoons of coconut oil
- 2 teaspoons of nutritional yeast
- 2 teaspoons of thyme
- 2 teaspoons of black pepper
- Sea salt

AAAAAAAAAAAAAAAAAAAAAA

Instruction:

A. In a mixing bowl, combine the tomato slices with black pepper, salt, thyme, coconut oil, and nutritional yeast. Ensure that the slices are evenly coated with the mixture.

B. Line a baking sheet with parchment paper for easy cleanup. Arrange the seasoned tomato slices on the parchment paper, making sure they are spread out in a single layer to allow even baking.

C. Preheat your oven to the recommended temperature, usually around 225°F to 250°F (107°C to 121°C). Place the baking sheet with the tomato slices in the preheated oven and bake them until they turn crisp. This typically takes around 2 to 3 hours. Keep a close eye on them to prevent over-browning.

D. Once the tomato slices have reached the desired level of crispness, carefully remove the baking sheet from the oven. Allow the tomato chips to cool down on the baking sheet for a few minutes. This helps them to become even crispier as they cool.

E. Transfer the cooled tomato chips to an airtight container. Ensure that the container is completely sealed to maintain their crisp texture. You can store them at room temperature for a few days, but for longer shelf life, keep them in the refrigerator.

F. When you're ready to enjoy your coconut-coated oven-baked tomato chips, simply grab a handful and savor the crispy, flavorful goodness. They make for a delightful and healthier snack option.

Cooking Notes:

- Experiment with the thickness of the tomato slices to achieve your preferred level of crispiness. Thinner slices will generally become crisper faster.
- Coconut oil adds a tropical flavor and healthy fats to the chips, enhancing both taste and texture.
- Tomato Selection: Choose ripe and firm tomatoes for optimal flavor and texture. Avoid overly ripe or mushy tomatoes, as they may not hold up well during the baking process.
- Salt Application: If you prefer a saltier flavor, you can sprinkle a bit of salt on the tomato slices before baking. Keep in mind that the nutritional yeast also adds a salty note to the chips.
- Thyme Variations: While thyme adds a lovely herbal note, you can experiment with other dried herbs such as oregano, rosemary, or basil to create different flavor profiles.
- Oven Rack Position: Place the baking sheet in the center or upper middle rack of the oven for even heat distribution. This helps the tomato slices bake uniformly.
- Checking for Crispness: The tomato chips will continue to crisp up as they cool. If you're unsure about their doneness, remove one slice from the oven and let it cool completely before testing its texture.
- Flavor Enhancements: For an extra layer of flavor, you can infuse the coconut oil with garlic or onion powder before tossing it with the tomato slices.
- Spice Options: Customize the flavor by adding a touch of cayenne pepper, smoked paprika, or a sprinkle of Italian seasoning to the tomato slices before baking.

- Storage Considerations: The airtight container is crucial for maintaining the crispiness of the chips. If you notice any moisture buildup inside the container, you can add a small piece of dry rice to help absorb excess moisture.
- Portion Control: While these tomato chips are healthier than many store-bought options, it's still a good idea to enjoy them in moderation due to their calorie content.
- Flavor Layering: Before baking, you can sprinkle some nutritional yeast on top of the tomato slices to create a cheese-like layer on the chips.
- Dipping Options: Serve the tomato chips with a side of hummus, guacamole, or a yogurt-based dip for added indulgence.
- Use for Garnish: Crumbled tomato chips can make a creative and flavorful garnish for soups, salads, or pasta dishes.
- Meal Component: Incorporate the tomato chips as a crunchy topping for sandwiches, wraps, or grain bowls to add both texture and a burst of flavor.
- Different Tomato Varieties: Experiment with different tomato varieties such as Roma, cherry, or grape tomatoes for unique shapes and flavors in your chips.
- Batch Size: Adjust the batch size based on your snacking needs. You can easily double or halve the recipe to suit your preferences.
- Fruit Leathers: You can also use the same approach to make tomato fruit leathers by blending the seasoned tomato mixture until smooth and spreading it thinly on a baking sheet lined with parchment paper. Dehydrate in the oven at a low temperature until dried but still pliable.
- Savory Breakfast Topping: Sprinkle the coconut-coated tomato chips on top of scrambled eggs or avocado toast for a savory and nutritious breakfast option.
- Gift Idea: Package these homemade tomato chips in decorative bags or containers as a unique and flavorful homemade gift for friends and family.

- Flavor Fusion: Create an international twist by adding spices like curry powder, garam masala, or za'atar to the tomato slices before baking for a global flavor experience.

- Nutritional yeast not only provides a cheesy and savory taste but also offers extra nutrients.

- Keep an eye on the baking time, as oven temperatures can vary. Adjust the baking time accordingly to prevent burning or undercooking.

- For added variety, consider sprinkling some grated Parmesan cheese or a touch of paprika before baking.

- To ensure maximum freshness, store these chips in an airtight container with a small piece of parchment paper to absorb excess moisture.

12. Spiced Poached Spanish Pear in Red Wine

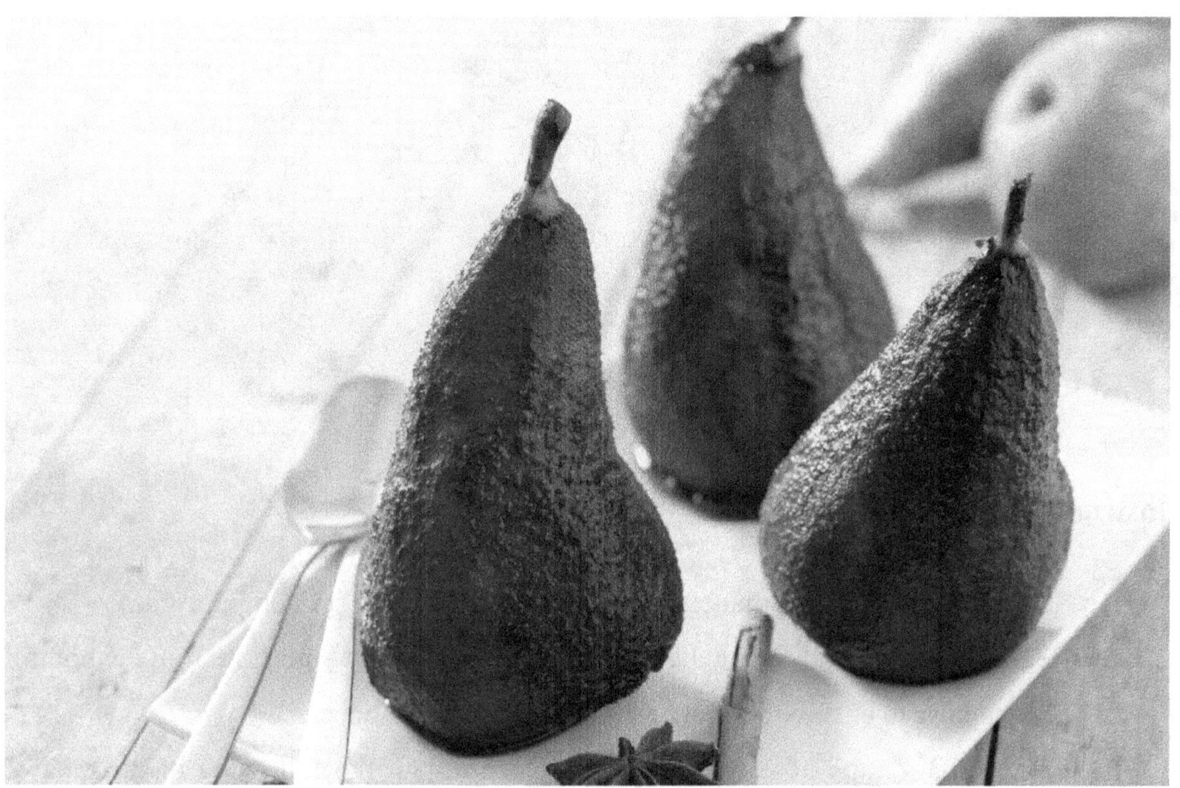

What could be a better combination than a glass of healthy flavonoids and fiber? You know what they say; a clean gut leads to a healthy exterior.

Duration: 80 minutes

Serving Size: 4

List of Ingredients:

- 4 large pears
- 2 sticks of cinnamon
- 6 to 10 cloves
- 2-star anise
- ½ cup of honey
- ½ an inch of ginger
- 1 vanilla pod
- 3 – 4 cups of red wine your choice

AAAAAAAAAAAAAAAAAAAA

Instruction:

A. Select a deep saucepan that can accommodate the pears standing upright.

B. Begin by peeling and coring the 4 large pears. Trim a small portion from the bottom of each pear to ensure they can stand upright in the saucepan.

C. Combine 3-4 cups of your choice of red wine with the following ingredients: 2 sticks of cinnamon, 6 to 10 cloves, 2-star anise, ½ cup of honey, half an inch of ginger (you can peel and slice it), and the seeds scraped from 1 vanilla pod.

D. Pour the prepared red wine mixture into the saucepan along with the cored and trimmed pears.

E. Place the saucepan on the stove and bring the mixture to a boil. Once it's boiling, reduce the heat to a gentle simmer.

F. Allow the pears to simmer in the liquid for approximately 30 to 40 minutes. You can test their doneness by inserting a knife into a pear – it should pierce through but still offer some firmness.

G. As the pears simmer, the liquid in the saucepan will naturally reduce by about half. This reduction will eventually become a flavorful sauce for the dish.

Cooking Notes:

- When choosing pears, opt for varieties that are suitable for poaching, such as Bosc or Bartlett. These varieties hold their shape well during cooking.
- You can adjust the amount of honey according to your sweetness preference.
- Make sure the saucepan is deep enough to fully submerge the pears in the liquid. This helps in even cooking and infusing flavors.
- Keep an eye on the simmering process to prevent the liquid from evaporating too quickly. Add more wine or water if needed to ensure the pears remain submerged.
- The cooking time might vary depending on the size and ripeness of the pears. Test their doneness by gently poking with a knife – they should be tender but not mushy.
- The reduced liquid serves as a delectable sauce to drizzle over the poached pears. Strain the liquid to remove the spices before serving.
- For an elegant presentation, serve the spiced poached pears with a spoonful of the reduced sauce and perhaps a dollop of whipped cream or a scoop of vanilla ice cream.

13. Mediterranean Nutty-sweet Saffron Rice

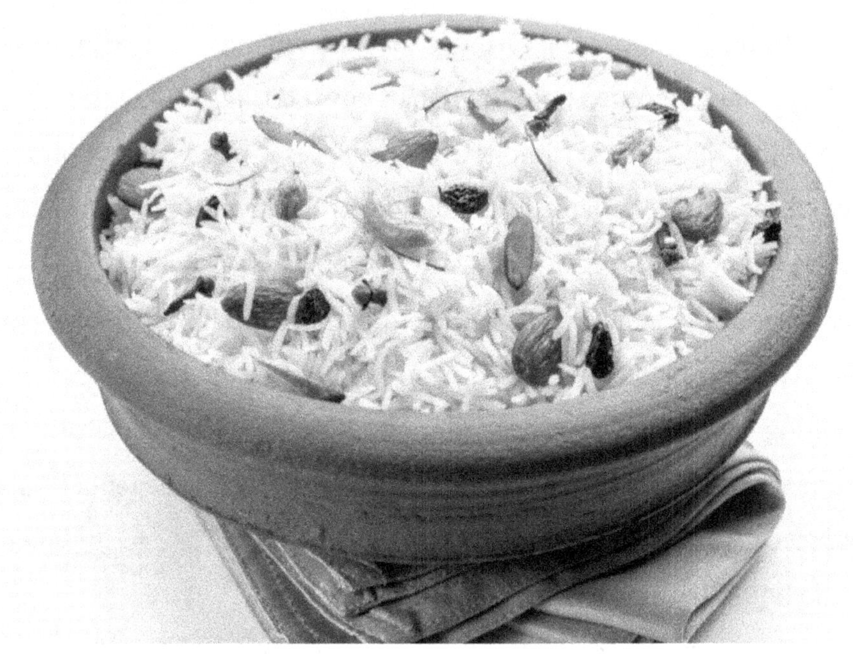

This powerful, bold flavor is packed with antioxidant that improves PMS and depression, factors of aging.

Duration: 35 minutes

Serving Size: 4-6

List of Ingredients:

- 2 cups of basmati or brown rice
- 2 stalks of mint with about 14 to 16 leaves
- 2 tablespoons of coconut oil or ghee or clarified butter
- 2 bay leaves
- 1 teaspoon of cardamom
- 1 stick of cinnamon
- 1 teaspoon or more of cumin
- 3 pinches of saffron
- 2 tablespoons of hot water
- 3 tablespoons of almond flakes
- ½ cup of pomegranate seed
- 3 tablespoons of roasted pistachio
- ¼ cup of dried raisin
- 4 cups of vegetable stock
- Salt and black pepper

AAAAAAAAAAAAAAAAAAAAAA

Instruction:

A. Begin by gently crushing the saffron threads and placing them in a small bowl. Pour hot water over the crushed saffron to rehydrate it. Set this saffron mixture aside.

B. In a saucepan, heat coconut oil over medium heat. Add bay leaves, cardamom pods, cinnamon sticks, and cumin seeds to the hot oil. Let them sizzle and release their aromatic flavors for about 1 minute.

C. Stir in the rice and let it toast in the fragrant oil and spices for about 2 minutes. This enhances the nutty flavor of the rice.

D. Pour in the rehydrated saffron mixture, along with the vegetable or chicken stock, and add the raisins. Season the mixture with salt and pepper to taste. Allow the rice to simmer and cook in the flavorful liquid. The saffron will infuse its golden color and distinctive taste into the rice.

E. Once the rice is cooked and has absorbed the liquid, remove the saucepan from the heat. Gently stir in the pistachio and almond flakes to add a delightful nutty crunch.

F. To finish the dish, garnish the Mediterranean nutty-sweet saffron rice with vibrant pomegranate seeds. These seeds add a burst of color, sweetness, and a juicy pop to every bite.

Cooking Notes:

- Handle saffron gently when crushing it, as it is delicate and can be quite expensive.
- Rehydrating saffron with hot water helps to release its flavor and color, enhancing the overall appeal of the dish.
- Toasting the rice with spices and oil before adding liquid can intensify the flavors of the rice and create a rich foundation for the dish.
- When adding stock, choose either vegetable or chicken stock based on your dietary preferences. This liquid will infuse the rice with a savory taste.
- The raisins add natural sweetness to the rice, complementing the saffron's unique flavor.
- When cooking the rice, follow the recommended time and liquid ratio on the rice packaging to ensure proper cooking.
- Quality Saffron Selection: Choose high-quality saffron threads to ensure the best flavor and color. Look for saffron that has a vibrant red color and a strong aroma.
- Saffron Water Infusion: Allow the saffron mixture to sit for a bit after adding hot water. This allows the saffron threads to release their color and flavor into the water.

- Spice Variation: Feel free to experiment with different whole spices like cloves, star anise, or fennel seeds to add depth and complexity to the rice.

- Liquid Measurement Accuracy: When adding stock, measure the liquid accurately to achieve the desired rice texture. Too much liquid can result in mushy rice, while too little can result in dry grains.

- Stock Temperature: Use warm or hot stock to maintain the temperature of the rice as it cooks and absorbs the liquid.

- Rinsing Rice: Rinse the rice under cold water before toasting it. This helps remove excess starch and prevents the rice from becoming overly sticky.

- Checking for Doneness: While cooking, check the rice for doneness by tasting a few grains. They should be tender but still have a slight firmness.

- Variety in Nut Options: Besides pistachios and almonds, consider using other nuts like cashews, pine nuts, or walnuts for additional texture and flavor.

- Flavorful Alternative: Instead of water, you can use chicken or vegetable broth to rehydrate the saffron. This adds even more flavor to the dish.

- Herb-Infused Oil: For an extra layer of flavor, infuse the coconut oil with herbs like rosemary or thyme before adding the rice.

- Colorful Veggie Addition: Incorporate finely chopped bell peppers or carrots to the rice for added color and nutrition.

- Nut Allergies: If you have nut allergies, you can omit the nuts or substitute them with toasted seeds like pumpkin seeds or sunflower seeds.

- Protein Pairing: Serve this saffron rice alongside grilled chicken, lamb, or fish for a complete and satisfying meal.

- Make-Ahead Tips: You can prepare the saffron mixture and spice-infused oil in advance. When ready to serve, reheat the oil, add the rice, and proceed with the recipe.

- Flavor Layering: For an added layer of complexity, sauté finely chopped onions or garlic before adding the rice to the saucepan.

- Pomegranate Alternative: If pomegranate seeds are not available, you can use dried cranberries or currants for a similar burst of sweetness and color.
- Serving Presentation: Layer the saffron rice on a serving platter and garnish it with a generous sprinkling of fresh herbs for a visually appealing presentation.
- Make It Creamy: To create a creamier texture, you can stir in a small amount of Greek yogurt or sour cream at the end of cooking.
- Leftover Reinvention: Use any leftover saffron rice to stuff bell peppers, zucchini, or tomatoes for a flavorful and creative dish.
- Cauliflower Rice Variation: For a low-carb option, you can substitute cauliflower rice for regular rice. Follow the same cooking steps but adjust the cooking time accordingly.
- Customized Seasoning: Adjust the amount of spices and seasoning to your taste preferences. Add more or less to create a flavor profile that suits you best.
- Stirring in pistachios and almond flakes at the end provides a satisfying crunch and additional layers of flavor.
- Pomegranate seeds not only provide a visual contrast but also offer a juicy and refreshing burst that balances the richness of the dish.
- This Mediterranean saffron rice can be served as a side dish or a main course, paired with grilled vegetables, meats, or seafood.
- Customize the dish by adding herbs like chopped fresh mint or parsley for a burst of freshness.

14. Spicy and Sweet Sesame Seed Brittle

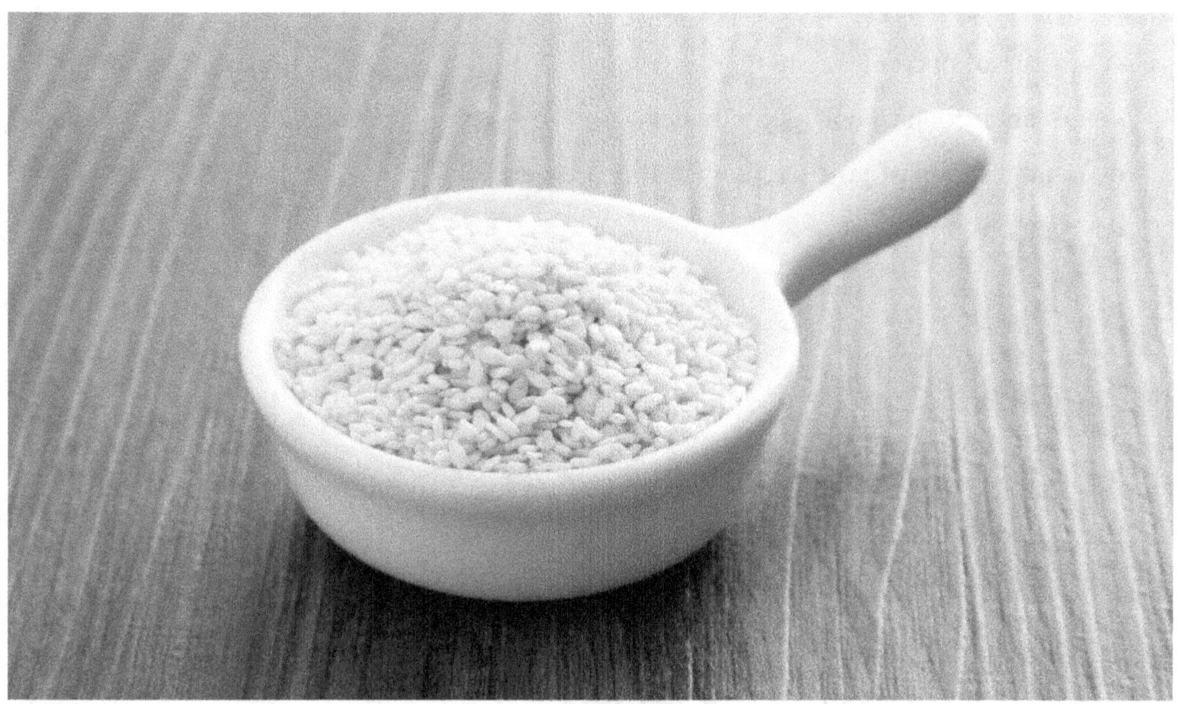

Maintain skin flexibility and elasticity with sesame seeds, and this is one way to snack healthily.

Duration: 15 minutes

Serving Size: 12 bars

List of Ingredients:

- 1 cup of sesame seeds
- ¾ cup of honey
- ¾ cup of coconut sugar
- ½ tablespoon of collagen powder
- 1 tablespoon of powdered crystalline ginger
- Salt

AAAAAAAAAAAAAAAAAAAAA

Instruction:

A. Start by placing a saucepan over medium heat. Combine honey, sugar, collagen powder, a pinch of salt, and grated ginger in the saucepan. Bring this mixture to a gentle simmer while stirring to ensure the ingredients dissolve and blend smoothly.

B. Once the mixture is well-simmered and the flavors are combined, add sesame seeds to the saucepan. Stir the mixture thoroughly until the sesame seeds are evenly coated and the mixture becomes thick.

C. To shape the brittle, place a silicone mat inside a bowl to create a mold. Pour the thickened sesame seed mixture onto the silicone mat. Use a spatula or the back of a spoon to spread and flatten the mixture, giving it the appearance of a bar.

D. Allow the mixture to cool and harden. Once it's completely cooled, carefully remove the sesame seed brittle from the silicone mat. Use a knife or your hands to cut the brittle into desired sizes or shapes.

E. Store the prepared spicy and sweet sesame seed brittle in an airtight container to maintain its freshness and crunch.

F. Now, you can enjoy your homemade spicy and sweet sesame seed brittle as a delicious treat.

Cooking Notes:

- When simmering the honey, sugar, collagen powder, salt, and ginger, be attentive to prevent the mixture from boiling over. Adjust the heat as needed to maintain a gentle simmer.
- Collagen powder might be included for nutritional benefits and texture. If preferred, you can omit it or substitute with other additives.
- When adding sesame seeds, make sure they are evenly distributed and well-coated with the syrup mixture. This ensures that each bite of the brittle has a balanced flavor and texture.
- Using a silicone mat in a bowl to mold the brittle allows you to shape it easily and gives it a neat appearance.
- Be cautious when cutting the cooled brittle, as it can be quite hard. Use a sharp knife and apply gentle pressure to avoid breaking it unevenly.
- Storing the brittle in an airtight container prevents moisture from affecting its texture and flavor. It also helps maintain its crispiness over time.
- Enjoy the sweet and spicy sesame seed brittle as a snack, dessert, or even as a topping for ice cream or yogurt.
- Experiment with the level of spiciness by adjusting the amount of grated ginger or adding a touch of chili powder or cayenne pepper for an extra kick.
- If you're concerned about the hard texture of the brittle, you can try adjusting the cooking time to achieve a chewier consistency. Keep in mind that altering the cooking time might affect the final texture and crunchiness.

15. Creamy Avocado Black Bean Salad

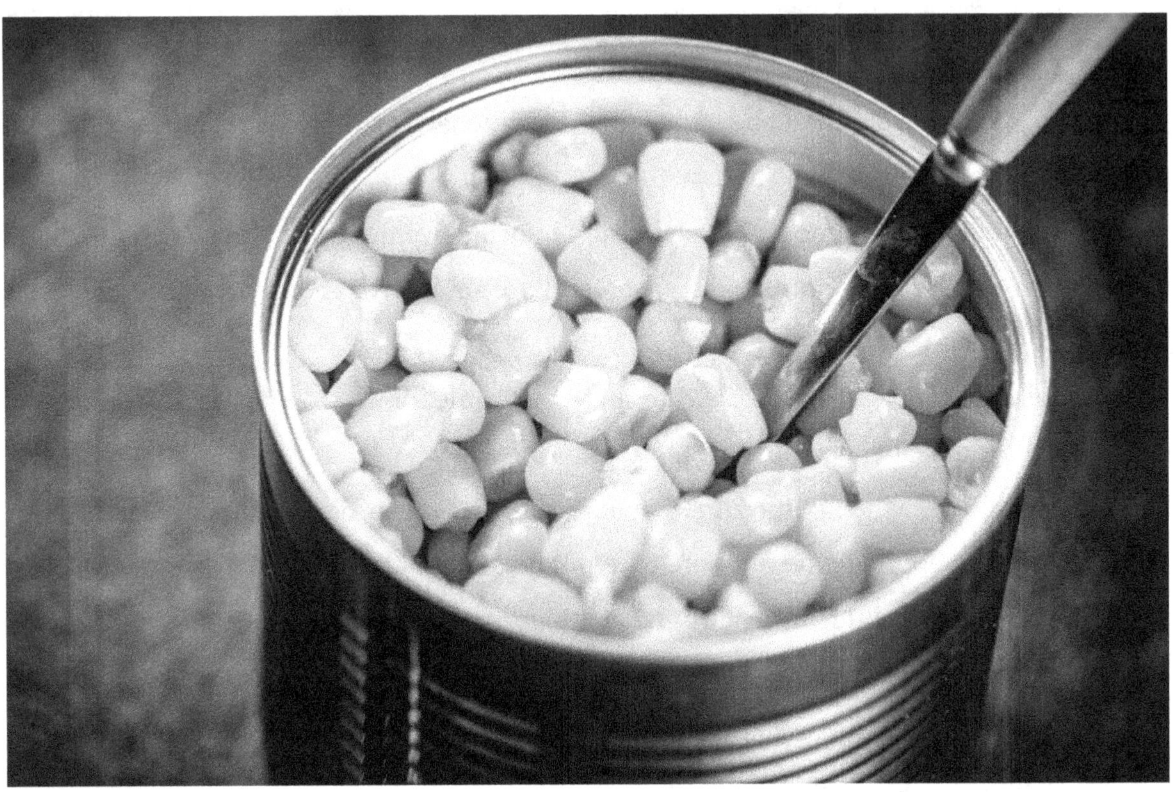

This plate of food is filled with a super healthy list of ingredients, fiber, and delicious nutrients to cleanse your system.

Duration: 12 – 15 minutes

Serving Size: 3

List of Ingredients:

- 2 cups of canned sweet corn drained
- 2 cups of canned black bean drained low sodium variety
- 1 cup of rehydrated dried sweet tomatoes sliced
- 1 small sweet white onion chopped
- 1 medium-size romaine lettuce about 4 cups
- 12 mint leaves chopped
- 1 avocado medium size
- 2 tablespoons of coconut cream
- 1 tablespoon of olive oil
- Salt and black pepper
- 1 lime, quartered

AAAAAAAAAAAAAAAAAAAAAA

Instruction:

A. Begin by preparing the creamy sauce. In a food processor, blend the medium-sized avocado, 2 tablespoons of coconut cream, 1 tablespoon of olive oil, and a pinch of salt and black pepper. Blend until you achieve a smooth and creamy consistency.

B. In a large bowl, combine the drained canned sweet corn, drained canned black beans (using the low-sodium variety), sliced rehydrated dried sweet tomatoes, chopped sweet white onion, and chopped mint leaves.

C. Pour the prepared creamy avocado sauce over the mixture in the large bowl. Gently toss and mix all the ingredients together until the sauce is evenly distributed and coats the salad ingredients.

D. Serve the creamy avocado black bean salad on a bed of medium-sized romaine lettuce leaves, which adds freshness and a crisp texture to the dish.

E. Garnish the salad with additional mint leaves for a burst of herbal aroma.

F. Serve the salad with lime quarters on the side. Squeezing lime over the salad before eating adds a zesty and refreshing flavor.

Cooking Notes:

- When blending the avocado for the creamy sauce, ensure it's ripe and soft for a smooth texture.
- Coconut cream provides creaminess and a touch of coconut flavor. You can adjust the quantity based on your preference.
- Using low-sodium canned black beans helps control the overall saltiness of the dish.
- Rehydrated dried sweet tomatoes add a chewy and intense tomato flavor to the salad. You can rehydrate them in warm water before slicing.
- Mint leaves contribute a refreshing and aromatic element to the salad. You can adjust the amount based on your taste preference.
- Romaine lettuce serves as a sturdy base for the salad and balances the creaminess of the avocado sauce.
- Squeezing lime over the salad before serving not only adds flavor but also enhances the overall taste profile of the dish.
- This creamy avocado black bean salad can be enjoyed as a light and refreshing meal on its own or as a side dish to complement other dishes.
- Feel free to customize the recipe by adding other ingredients like diced bell peppers, diced cucumber, or chopped cilantro for added color and flavor.
- If you're serving the salad later, consider keeping the creamy avocado sauce separate until just before serving to maintain the freshness of the ingredients.
- Adjust the seasoning and lime juice according to your taste preferences. Some extra lime juice can brighten up the flavors of the salad.

16. Summer Time Eucalyptus Green Tea

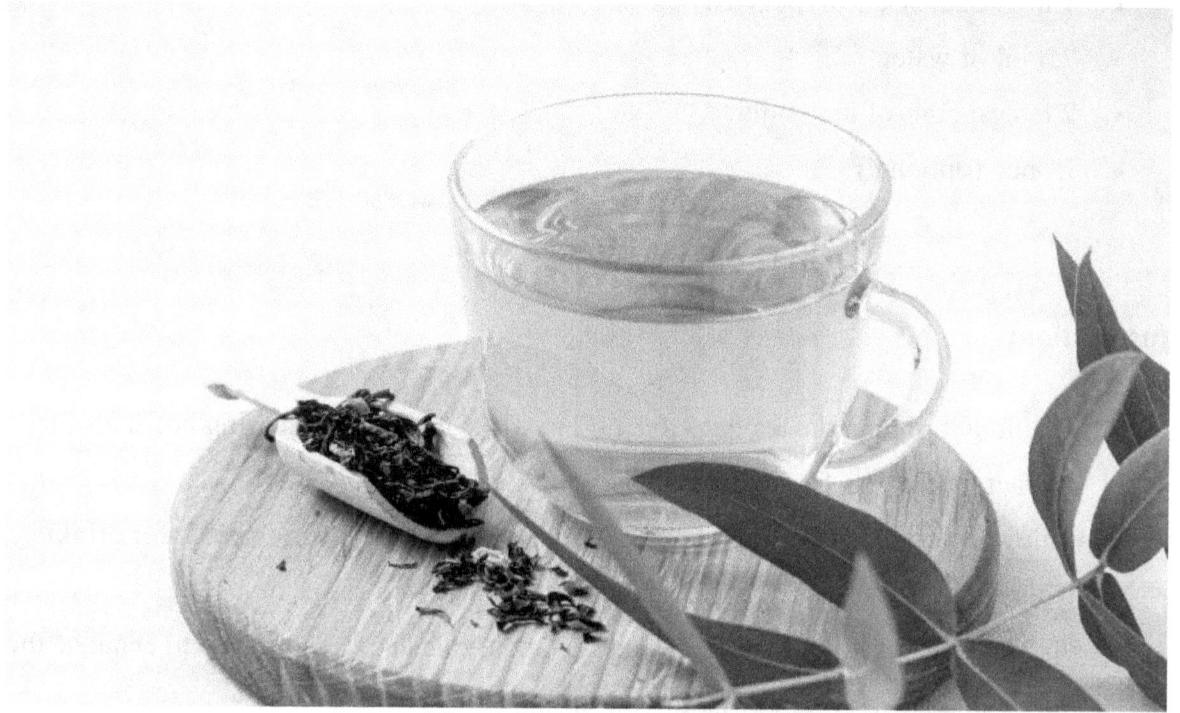

Keep your cells healthy and your body free of toxins with this green tea recipe. The eucalyptus is a great way to snooze unhindered.

Duration: 10 minutes

Serving Size: 2

List of Ingredients:

- 2 high-quality green tea bags
- 1 high-quality eucalyptus tea bag
- 750ml of water
- 2 tablespoons of lemon juice
- Honey (optional)

AAAAAAAAAAAAAAAAAAAAA

Instruction:

A. Begin by bringing the tea bags to a boil in water until it's simmering hot. This helps extract the flavors from the tea bags.

B. Allow the boiled tea to cool down to a temperature that is comfortable for drinking. This cooling process lets the tea reach a drinkable and refreshing state.

C. Just before you're ready to enjoy the tea, add a splash of lemon juice to enhance the flavor and add a citrusy twist to your drink.

D. If you prefer a touch of sweetness, you can add honey to the tea. This adds natural sweetness and balances the flavors.

E. Now, you're all set to enjoy your Summer Time Eucalyptus Green Tea. Sip and savor the refreshing and soothing qualities of the drink.

Cooking Notes:

- Use high-quality green tea bags for the best flavor. Eucalyptus-infused green tea can add a unique twist, but regular green tea works well too.
- Boiling the tea bags ensures that the tea releases its flavors and beneficial compounds. However, avoid over-boiling, as it can make the tea bitter.
- Cooling the tea is important to make it enjoyable to drink. If you're in a hurry, you can speed up the cooling process by placing the tea in the refrigerator.
- Adding lemon juice just before consumption preserves the freshness of the citrus flavor. Lemon also offers a burst of vitamin C.
- When adding honey, consider using raw or organic honey for its natural sweetness and potential health benefits.
- Customize the sweetness level and lemon flavor to match your taste preferences.
- Eucalyptus green tea can have a mild herbal and slightly minty taste, which can be refreshing and soothing, especially during the summer months.
- Consider experimenting with other herbs or fruits for added complexity and flavor to your green tea.
- Keep in mind that consuming large amounts of eucalyptus or any herb may have potential health effects, so moderation is key.
- If you're making iced tea, let it cool completely before adding ice to avoid dilution.
- Green tea does contain caffeine, so be mindful of your caffeine intake if you're sensitive to it or plan to consume the tea later in the day.
- Remember to consult your healthcare professional if you have any medical conditions or concerns before making significant changes to your diet, including herbal teas.

17. It's just Poached Eggs

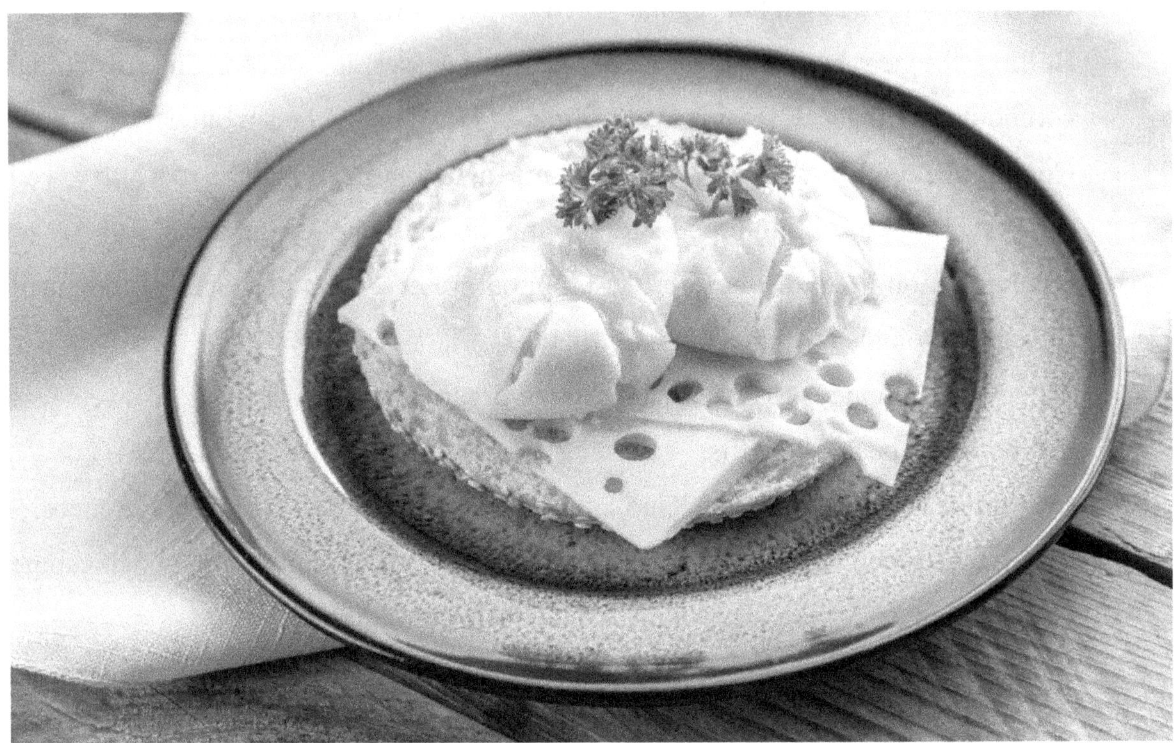

Well, that was what we thought, but there is more to eggs. It is nutrient-filled and a great way to boost collagen.

Duration: 20 minutes

Serving Size: 1

List of Ingredients:

- 2 large eggs
- 2 tablespoons of white vinegar
- ½ teaspoon of chili flakes
- Kosher salt to taste

AAAAAAAAAAAAAAAAAAAAA

Instruction:

A. Start by bringing a large pot of water to a gentle boil. Add a splash of vinegar to the boiling water. The vinegar helps the egg white coagulate more effectively during poaching.

B. Crack an egg into a bowl, taking care not to break the yolk. This step helps ensure that the egg is ready to be added to the water.

C. Use a spoon to gently stir the boiling water, creating a gentle whirlpool effect. This swirling motion helps the egg white wrap around the yolk as you poach it.

D. While the water is still swirling, carefully pour the cracked egg into the center of the whirlpool. The swirling water will help the egg white envelop the yolk for a classic poached egg shape.

E. Allow the egg to cook in the gently simmering water until it reaches the desired doneness. This can take around 3 to 4 minutes for a runny yolk, or a bit longer for a firmer yolk.

F. Once the egg is cooked to your liking, use a slotted spoon to carefully lift it out of the water. Gently drain any excess water from the spoon before placing the poached egg on a plate.

G. If desired, sprinkle a dash of salt and pepper over the poached egg to enhance its flavor.

H. Repeat the process for as many eggs as you'd like to poach.

I. Now, your perfectly poached eggs are ready to be enjoyed. The soft, runny yolk pairs well with a variety of dishes.

Cooking Notes:

- Adding vinegar to the boiling water helps coagulate the egg white more efficiently, resulting in a neater poached egg.
- Crack the egg into a bowl first to ensure that the yolk remains intact and to easily slide it into the water.
- Stirring the water before adding the egg creates a swirling motion that assists in shaping the egg as it poaches.
- Water that is too vigorously boiling can break up the egg and create a mess. Maintain a gentle simmer for best results.
- Poaching times can vary depending on the size of the egg and personal preference. Adjust the timing to achieve the desired yolk consistency.
- To achieve a runny yolk, a 3- to 4-minute cooking time is a good starting point. Adjust this time for softer or firmer yolks.
- Using a slotted spoon to lift the poached egg out of the water helps drain excess water and prevents the egg from becoming waterlogged.
- Serve the poached eggs on their own, over toast, with sautéed vegetables, or as part of a delicious eggs Benedict.
- Be sure to use fresh eggs for poaching, as fresher eggs have a thicker egg white that holds its shape better during cooking.
- Experiment with adding a splash of white wine or a touch of lemon juice to the poaching water for additional flavor variations.
- Poached eggs can be enjoyed as a wholesome and protein-rich meal, and they are also a versatile component in various dishes.

18. Sweet Chocolate Chips Oatmeal Muffin

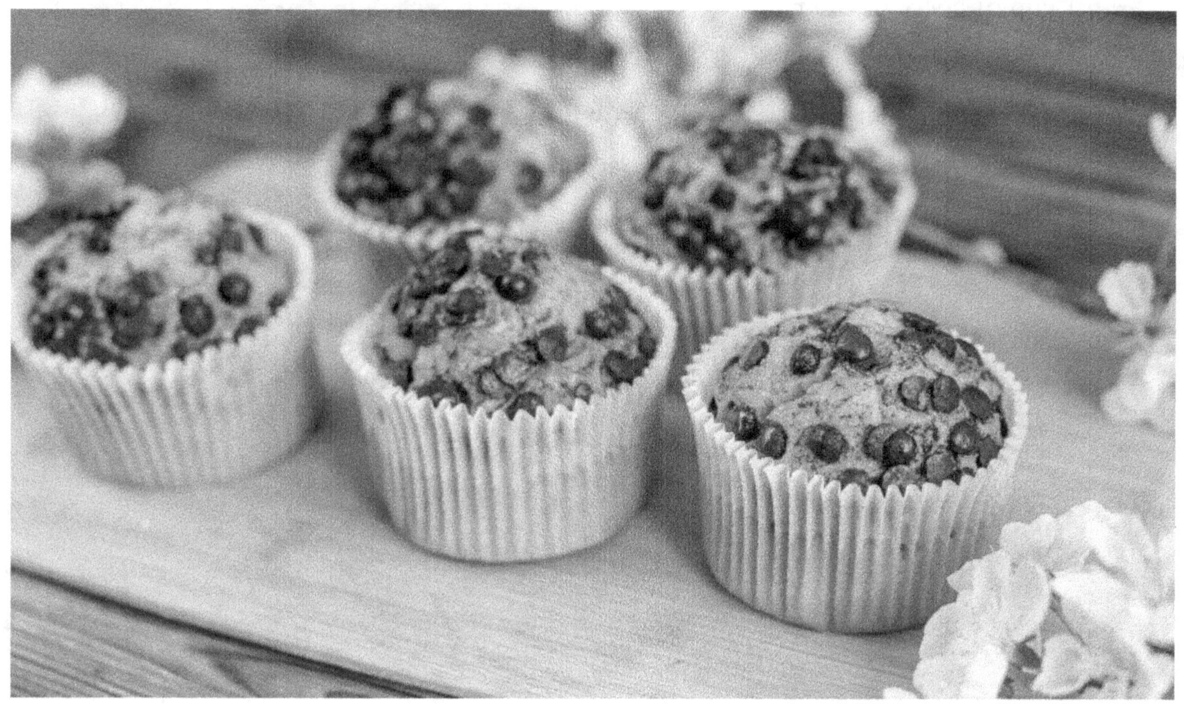

Oatmeal is a feel-happy food that is super satisfying. If you are happy, you feel and look younger.

Duration: 25 minutes

Serving Size: 12 muffin

List of Ingredients:

- ½ cup of wheat flour
- 1 cup of coconut flour
- 1 cup of rolled oats
- ½ cup of coconut sugar or ¼ cup brown sugar
- 1 baking powder
- ½ teaspoon of baking soda
- 3 eggs
- 2 large bananas
- ½ cup of coconut milk
- ¾ cup of milk chocolate chips
- ½ teaspoon of Kosher salt
- ½ cup of oats extra

AAAAAAAAAAAAAAAAAAAAA

Instruction:

A. Start by preheating your oven to the specified temperature. Then, line a baking tray with large muffin papers to prepare for baking.

B. Begin by mixing the dry ingredients together in a bowl. Combine ½ cup of wheat flour, 1 cup of coconut flour, 1 cup of rolled oats, coconut sugar (or brown sugar), baking powder, baking soda, and ½ teaspoon of Kosher salt. Once combined, set this dry mixture aside.

C. In another bowl, mix the wet ingredients. Mash 2 large bananas and beat in 3 eggs. Add ½ cup of coconut milk to the mixture, along with the milk chocolate chips. Ensure the wet ingredients are well combined.

D. Combine the wet mixture with the dry mixture by adding the wet ingredients into the bowl with the dry ingredients. Gently mix the two together until just combined. Be careful not to overmix, as this can affect the texture of the muffins.

E. After combining the wet and dry ingredients, fold in the milk chocolate chips to evenly distribute them throughout the batter.

F. For an added crunch, sprinkle extra oats over the top of the batter. This not only adds texture but also enhances the appearance of the muffins.

G. Pour the muffin batter into the lined muffin papers in the baking tray. Distribute the batter evenly among the muffin cups.

H. Place the tray in the preheated oven and bake the muffins until they are fully cooked and golden brown. Baking time may vary, but it usually takes around 15-20 minutes.

I. Once the muffins are baked and have a golden appearance, remove them from the oven and let them cool slightly.

J. Now, you're ready to enjoy your Sweet Chocolate Chips Oatmeal Muffins. These delightful treats are perfect for satisfying your sweet tooth in a healthier way.

Cooking Notes:

- Preheating the oven ensures that the muffins bake at the right temperature, promoting even cooking and proper rise.
- Using muffin papers prevents the muffins from sticking to the tray and makes them easier to handle after baking.
- Coconut flour and rolled oats contribute to the nutritional value and texture of the muffins.
- The choice between coconut sugar and brown sugar affects the sweetness and flavor profile of the muffins.

- Mixing wet and dry ingredients separately before combining them helps ensure even distribution of ingredients.

- Adding bananas to the wet mixture enhances sweetness and contributes to the muffins' moistness.

- Folding in the chocolate chips prevents over mixing and uneven distribution of the chips.

- Sprinkling extra oats on top before baking provides visual appeal and a satisfying crunch.

- Be vigilant while baking to prevent overcooking, which can result in dry muffins.

- Allow the muffins to cool slightly before enjoying them, as they will be easier to handle and the flavors will have time to settle.

- These muffins can be stored in an airtight container for a few days, but their freshness is best on the day of baking.

- Feel free to adjust the sweetness level and the quantity of chocolate chips to suit your taste preferences.

- If you're making these muffins for your dog, ensure that all ingredients are safe and suitable for canine consumption.

19. Spinach & Quinoa Stuffed Button Mushrooms

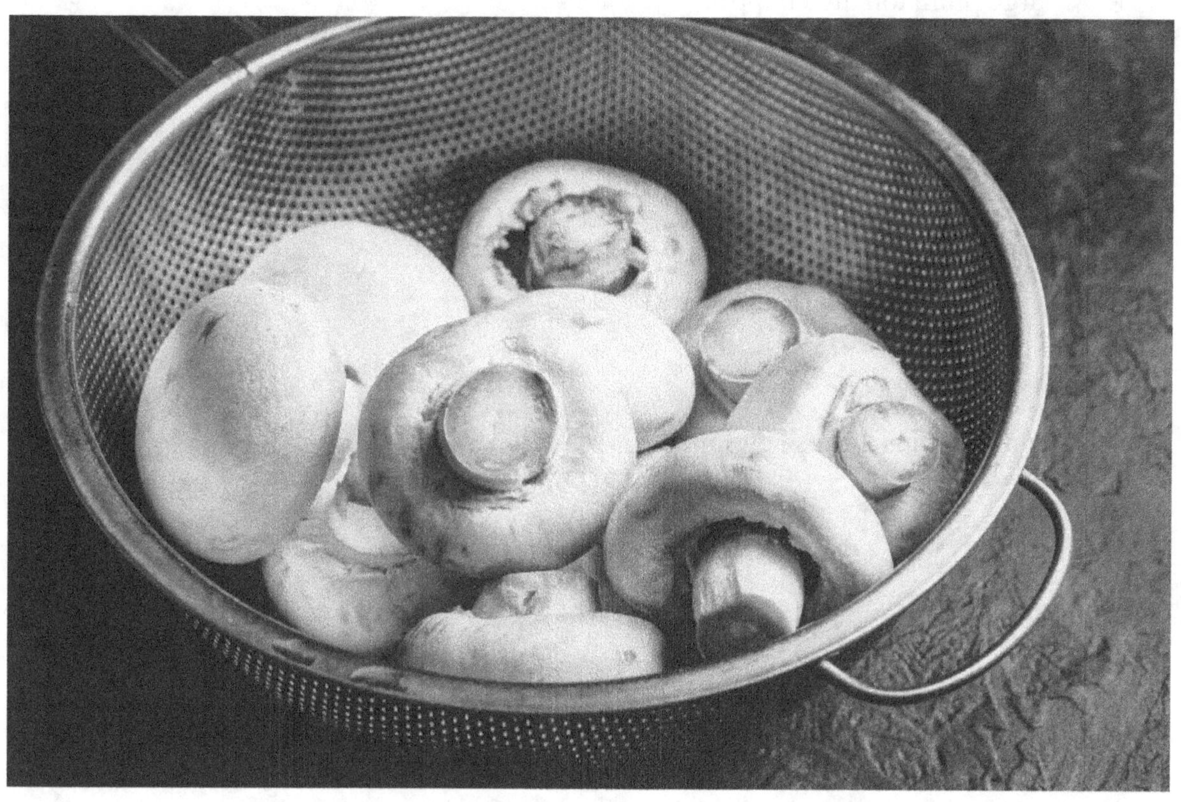

The first signs of aging are achy bones, joints, and deformed structures. Mushrooms contain Vitamin D and enable your body to get all the calcium for bone health.

Bake Temp 375 F

Duration: 22 minutes

Serving Size: 4

List of Ingredients:

- 16 button mushrooms, cleaned with a kitchen towel
- 1 cup of partially cooked quinoa
- 1 tablespoon of light soy sauce
- 1 large plum tomato chopped
- 1 small onion chopped
- 1 teaspoon of minced garlic
- 1 small chili chopped
- 1 cup of crumbled goat cheese
- 2 stalk scallions chopped
- 1 – 2 tablespoons of olive oil
- Salt and black pepper
- 2 cups of spinach fresh chopped

AAAAAAAAAAAAAAAAAAAAAA

Instruction:

A. Begin by removing the stalks from the button mushrooms, creating a hollow space for the stuffing.

B. In a bowl, combine the partially cooked quinoa, chopped plum tomato, chopped onion, minced garlic, chopped chili, crumbled goat cheese, chopped scallions, and fresh chopped spinach. Season the mixture with light soy sauce, salt, and black pepper. Mix the ingredients thoroughly to ensure even distribution of flavors.

C. Using spoonfuls of the prepared stuffing mixture, neatly fill the hollowed mushrooms with the mixture. Make sure to evenly distribute the stuffing among all the mushrooms.

D. Place the stuffed mushrooms on a baking tray, arranging them neatly to avoid overcrowding.

E. Preheat your oven to the specified temperature. Check the mushrooms after about 10 minutes of baking and, if needed, reduce the oven temperature to 275°F (135°C) to finish cooking. The total baking time may vary, but the mushrooms should be cooked until they are tender and the filling is heated through.

F. Once the mushrooms are cooked to your liking, remove them from the oven. Allow them to cool slightly before serving.

Cooking Notes:

- Cleaning the button mushrooms with a kitchen towel helps remove any dirt or debris from the surface.
- Partially cooking the quinoa beforehand ensures that it is fully cooked and tender once the stuffed mushrooms are baked.
- Light soy sauce adds a savory umami flavor to the stuffing mixture. Adjust the amount based on your taste preferences.
- Chopped plum tomato, onion, minced garlic, and chili contribute to the flavor profile of the stuffing mixture.
- Crumbled goat cheese provides creaminess and tanginess to the stuffing. You can substitute it with other cheeses if desired.
- Chopped scallions add a mild onion flavor and a touch of freshness to the stuffing mixture.
- Fresh chopped spinach not only adds color but also provides nutrients and a slight earthy taste.
- Carefully spooning the stuffing into the mushrooms ensures that each mushroom is properly filled and looks appealing.

- Baking the stuffed mushrooms at a higher temperature initially helps them cook and develop a nice crust, while lowering the temperature towards the end prevents overcooking or burning.

- The stuffed mushrooms are ready when the mushrooms are tender and the stuffing is heated through.

- These stuffed mushrooms can be served as an appetizer, side dish, or even a light main course.

- Consider garnishing the stuffed mushrooms with additional chopped herbs like parsley or basil before serving.

- Keep in mind that mushrooms tend to release moisture as they cook, so the baking tray may accumulate some liquid. Be cautious when handling the tray after baking.

- If serving these stuffed mushrooms to guests, you can sprinkle a little extra crumbled goat cheese or herbs on top for a finishing touch.

- Always ensure that any ingredients used are safe and suitable for your dietary preferences and any dietary restrictions you might have.

- If making these for a specific audience (such as dogs), ensure that all ingredients are safe and appropriate for that audience's consumption.

20. Simple Garlic Pan Steamed Spinach

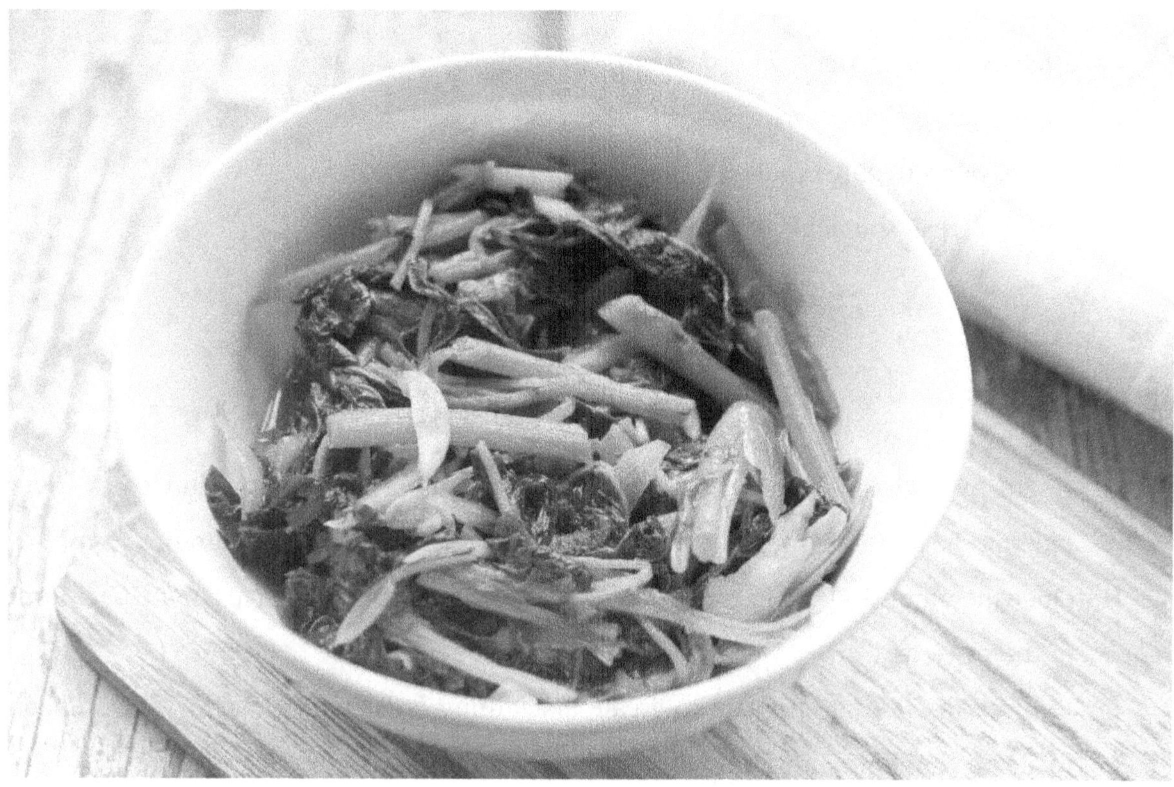

Spinach is loaded with a lot of goodies and components that help improve skin texture and elasticity.

Duration: 10 minutes

Serving Size: 3

List of Ingredients:

- 2 tablespoons of chicken stock
- 2 cloves of garlic, thinly sliced
- 2 tablespoons of finely chopped onion
- 1 tablespoon of extra virgin olive oil
- Sea salt and freshly cracked peppercorn
- 600g of fresh spinach

AAAAAAAAAAAAAAAAAAAAA

Instruction:

A. Begin by adding oil to a non-stick pan and sautéing the onion and garlic over medium heat. Sauté until the onion and garlic become soft and fragrant.

B. Once the onion and garlic are softened, add the fresh spinach leaves to the pan. Pour in the stock as well.

C. Replace the lid onto the pan to create a steaming environment. Allow the spinach to steam for about 3 to 5 minutes, or until it wilts and becomes tender.

D. Once the spinach is steamed to your desired level of doneness, remove the lid from the pan.

E. Serve the Simple Garlic Pan Steamed Spinach, seasoning it with salt and pepper according to your taste preferences.

Cooking Notes:

- Using a non-stick pan helps prevent the spinach from sticking to the pan during sautéing and steaming.
- Sautéing the onion and garlic in oil releases their flavors and aromas, adding depth to the dish.
- Adding stock to the pan creates steam, which helps wilt and cook the spinach.
- The lid is used to trap steam and heat, which accelerates the steaming process and ensures even cooking.
- Steaming spinach preserves its vibrant green color and many of its nutrients.
- The cooking time for steaming spinach is relatively short, as it doesn't require extended cooking to become tender.
- Seasoning the dish with salt and pepper at the end enhances the flavors of the spinach and complements the garlic and onion.
- This simple dish can be served as a nutritious side or added to various dishes, such as pasta, rice, or protein.
- Customize the dish by adding additional seasonings or ingredients like lemon juice, red pepper flakes, or grated cheese.
- Always ensure that any ingredients used are safe and suitable for your dietary preferences and any dietary restrictions you might have.
- If you're making this dish for dogs, ensure that all ingredients are safe and appropriate for canine consumption, and consider their individual dietary needs and sensitivities.

21. Creamy Avocado Hummus

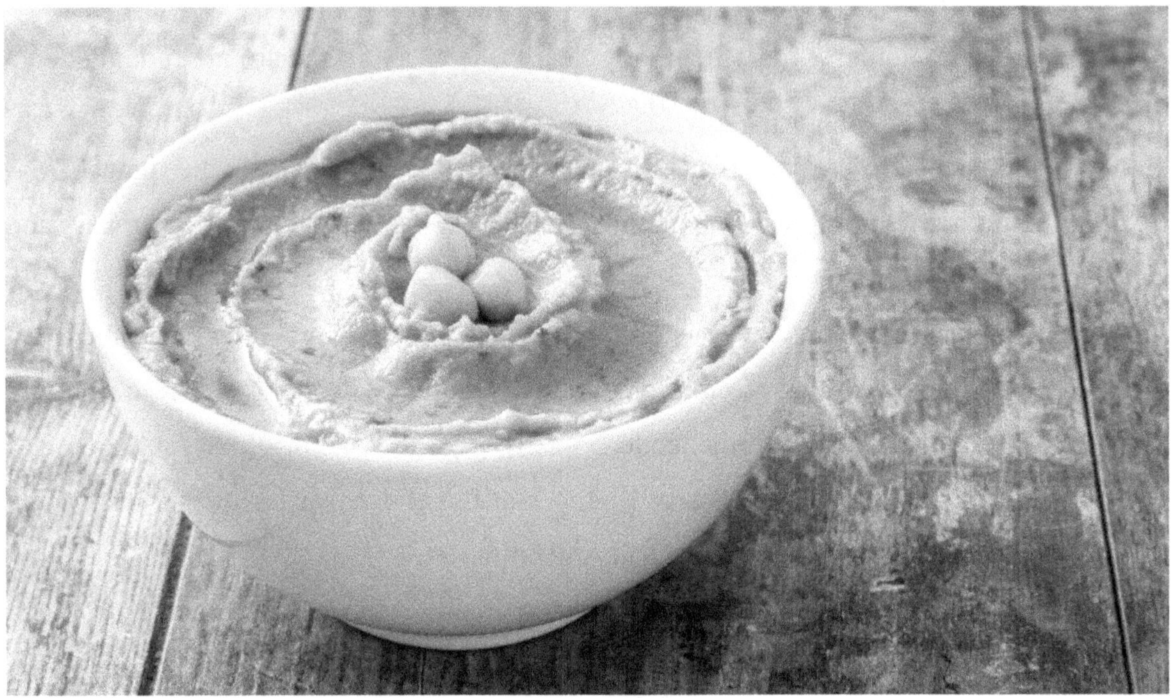

Full of omega-3s, avocados are jam-packed with anti-inflammatory and immune-boosting properties, and if you like hummus, this is a healthier way to go.

Duration: 10 minutes

Serving Size: 6 – 8

List of Ingredients:

- 1 ½ cups of chickpeas soaked overnight
- 1 large avocado or 2 cups equivalent
- ¼ cup of sesame paste – tahini
- 1 large lime
- ¼ teaspoon of cumin powder
- 6 mint leaves
- 3 tablespoons of olive oil
- ½ teaspoon of chili flakes
- A dash of salt as desired

AAAAAAAAAAAAAAAAAAAAAA

Instruction:

A. Begin by placing the soaked chickpeas, large avocado (or equivalent amount), sesame paste (tahini), juice of a large lime, cumin powder, mint leaves, and olive oil in a food processor.
B. Process all the ingredients in the food processor until they form a smooth and creamy mixture. The combination of chickpeas, avocado, and tahini creates a rich and velvety texture.
C. Once the creamy mixture is well blended, transfer it into a bowl. Next, add the remaining olive oil and sprinkle in the chili flakes. Season the mixture with a dash of salt, adjusting to your taste preferences.

Cooking Notes:

- Soaking the chickpeas overnight is essential to ensure they are softened and ready for blending. This step helps achieve a smoother hummus texture.

- Using a food processor facilitates the blending of the ingredients and creates a homogeneous mixture.
- The combination of chickpeas and avocado adds creaminess and a boost of nutrients to the hummus.
- Sesame paste (tahini) contributes to the classic flavor profile of hummus and enhances its texture.
- Fresh lime juice adds a zesty and tangy element to the hummus, balancing the flavors.
- Mint leaves infuse a refreshing and aromatic note into the hummus, complementing the other ingredients.
- Adding olive oil both during processing and as a finishing touch contributes to the hummus's smoothness and flavor.
- Chili flakes provide a subtle kick of heat to the hummus. Adjust the amount based on your spice preference.
- Seasoning the hummus with salt is important to enhance the overall taste and bring out the flavors of the ingredients.
- This creamy avocado hummus can be served as a dip with vegetables, pita bread, or crackers. It can also be used as a spread in sandwiches or wraps.
- Customize the hummus by adding additional ingredients such as roasted garlic, roasted red pepper, or different herbs for flavor variations.
- Storing the hummus in an airtight container in the refrigerator helps maintain its freshness and flavor.
- Always ensure that any ingredients used are safe and suitable for your dietary preferences and any dietary restrictions you might have.
- If you're making this hummus for dogs, ensure that all ingredients are safe and appropriate for canine consumption, and consider their individual dietary needs and sensitivities. Consulting with a veterinarian can be helpful in ensuring the hummus is suitable for your dog.

22. Sweet, Spicy, & Sour Edamame Snack

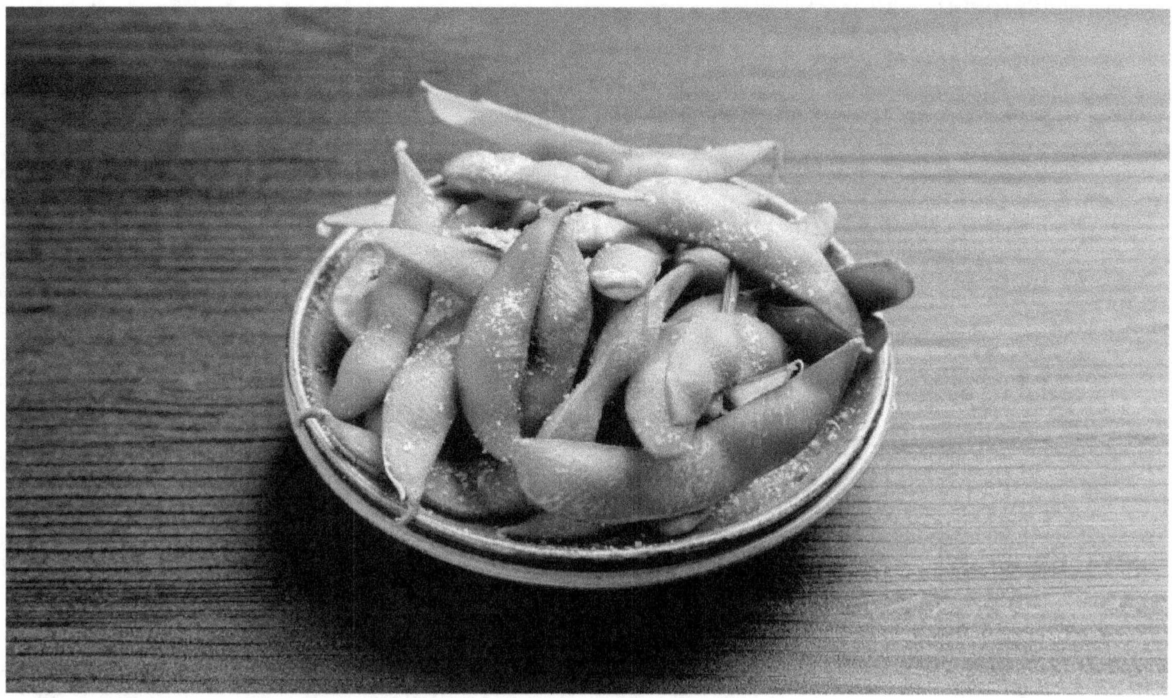

Health worries are the biggest cause of aging in women, but if your health is fine, aging disappears. Edamame boosts bone and heart health, and it tastes delicious too.

Duration: 10 minutes

Serving Size: 2

List of Ingredients:

- 500g of fresh edamame
- 1 teaspoon of minced garlic
- 1-inch piece of ginger, grated
- 1 small green chili, chopped
- 1 tablespoon of balsamic vinegar
- 1 teaspoon of tamarind paste
- 1 tablespoon of cane sugar
- Salt and pepper
- 1 tablespoon of rice bran oil

AAAAAAAAAAAAAAAAAAAAA

Instruction:

A. Start by rinsing the edamame thoroughly to remove any dirt or debris. Boil the edamame in water for about 3 to 5 minutes until they become bright green. This quick boiling process not only cooks the edamame but also enhances their vibrant green color.

B. After boiling, immediately transfer the boiled edamame to a bowl of cold water and let them soak for about 1 minute. This helps stop the cooking process and ensures that the edamame retains its crisp texture.

C. In a saucepan, add rice oil and heat it up. Sauté minced garlic, grated ginger, chopped chili, and tamarind paste in the heated oil. These ingredients will infuse the dish with a combination of sweet, spicy, and sour flavors.

D. Once the sautéed mixture is aromatic and well combined, add cane sugar and seasonings to balance the flavors. The combination of sweet and savory elements enhances the overall taste of the dish.

E. Toss the blanched and drained edamame into the saucepan with the sautéed mixture. Make sure the edamame is well coated with the flavorful mixture.

F. Finish the dish by drizzling balsamic vinegar over the edamame. The balsamic vinegar adds a tangy depth of flavor that compliments the other taste elements.

G. Serve the Sweet, Spicy, & Sour Edamame Snack as a flavorful and satisfying treat.

Cooking Notes:

- Boiling the edamame briefly in boiling water enhances their color and helps soften them slightly for easier eating.

- Soaking the boiled edamame in cold water immediately after boiling helps retain their vibrant color and prevents overcooking.

- Sautéing garlic, ginger, chili, and tamarind paste in rice oil creates a fragrant and flavorful base for the dish.

- Tamarind paste adds a tangy and sour note to the dish, balancing the sweetness and spice.

- Cane sugar balances the flavors by adding sweetness to contrast with the other taste elements.

- The choice of chili can be adjusted based on your desired level of spiciness.

- Adding seasonings and balancing the flavors is essential to achieving a harmonious taste profile.

- Drizzling balsamic vinegar at the end adds a final layer of flavor that ties everything together.

- This edamame snack can be served as a side dish, appetizer, or even a healthy snack option.

- Always ensure that any ingredients used are safe and suitable for your dietary preferences and any dietary restrictions you might have.

- If you're making this snack for dogs, ensure that all ingredients are safe and appropriate for canine consumption, and consider their individual dietary needs and sensitivities. Consulting with a veterinarian can be helpful in ensuring the snack is suitable for your dog.

23. Nutty Fruity Frozen Yogurt

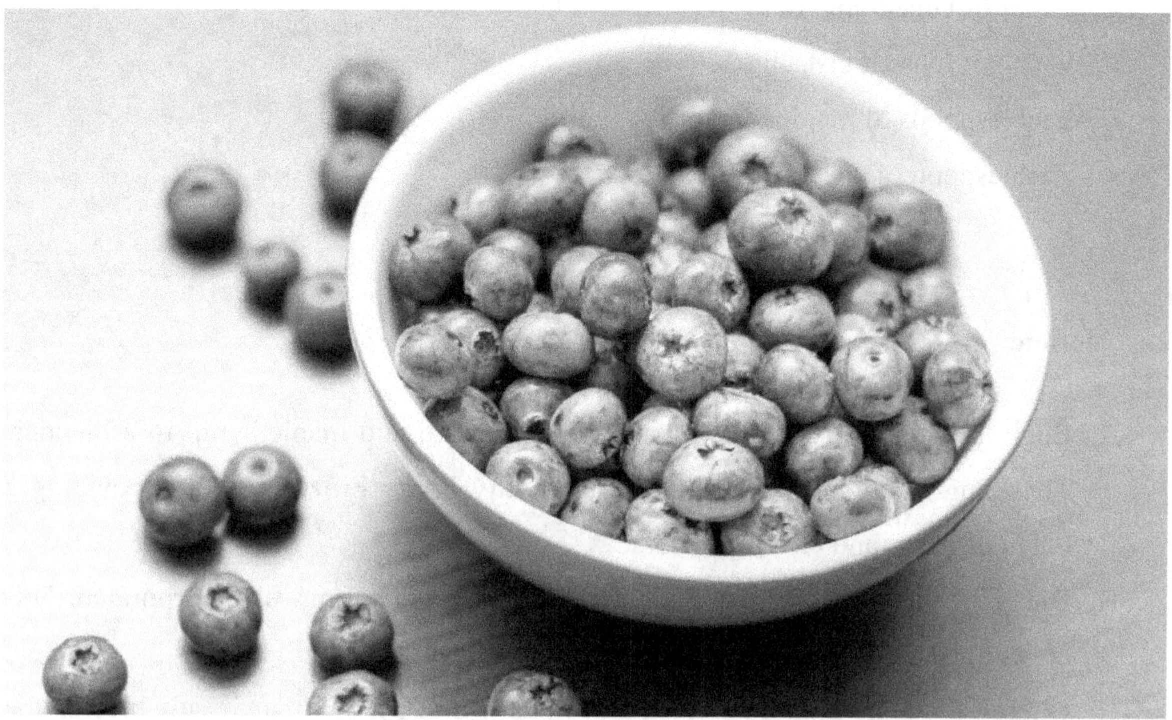

Yogurt keeps your cells young and healthy. Healthy cells, healthy you and this recipe contains all the good things you need.

Duration: 10 minutes

Serving Size: 4

List of Ingredients:

- 3 cups of fresh blueberries
- 1 liter of Greek yogurt
- ½ cup of toasted pistachio
- 2 tablespoons of maple syrup
- 1 tablespoon of coconut flakes

AAAAAAAAAAAAAAAAAAAAA

Instruction:

A. Begin by adding fresh blueberries, Greek yogurt, and maple syrup to a blender. These ingredients form the base of the Nutty Fruity Frozen Yogurt, providing a blend of fruity and creamy flavors.

B. Blend the mixture in the blender until all the ingredients are well incorporated. This creates a smooth and flavorful yogurt mixture that will freeze nicely.

C. Once the yogurt mixture is blended, pour it into a bowl that is suitable for the freezer. The bowl should be freezer-safe to ensure the yogurt sets properly.

D. Before freezing the yogurt mixture, sprinkle the toasted pistachios and coconut flakes over the top. These add a delightful nutty and tropical crunch to the frozen yogurt.

E. Place the bowl with the yogurt mixture in the freezer. Allow it to freeze for several hours until it reaches a firm and scoopable consistency.

F. When serving, scoop the Nutty Fruity Frozen Yogurt into bowls or cones. The combination of creamy yogurt, sweet blueberries, crunchy pistachios, and coconut flakes offers a delicious and refreshing treat.

Cooking Notes:

- Using fresh blueberries adds natural sweetness and a vibrant color to the frozen yogurt.
- Greek yogurt provides a creamy and tangy base for the frozen yogurt, offering a higher protein content compared to regular yogurt.
- Maple syrup enhances the sweetness of the frozen yogurt while adding a hint of natural flavor.
- Toasted pistachios contribute a satisfying crunch and nutty flavor to the dessert.
- Coconut flakes provide a tropical touch and an additional layer of texture to the frozen yogurt.
- Ensure the bowl you use for freezing is freezer-safe and can accommodate the yogurt mixture without overflowing.
- Allow the frozen yogurt to set in the freezer for several hours, ideally overnight, to achieve a solid and scoopable texture.
- When serving, consider garnishing with extra fresh blueberries, mint leaves, or other desired toppings.
- Homemade frozen yogurt is a versatile treat that can be customized with different fruits, nuts, and flavors to suit your taste preferences.
- Always ensure that any ingredients used are safe and suitable for your dietary preferences and any dietary restrictions you might have.
- If you're making this frozen yogurt for dogs, ensure that all ingredients are safe and appropriate for canine consumption, and consider their individual dietary needs and sensitivities. Consulting with a veterinarian can be helpful in ensuring the frozen yogurt is suitable for your dog.

24. Ghee Sautéed Shrimp with Creamy Cilantro Sauce

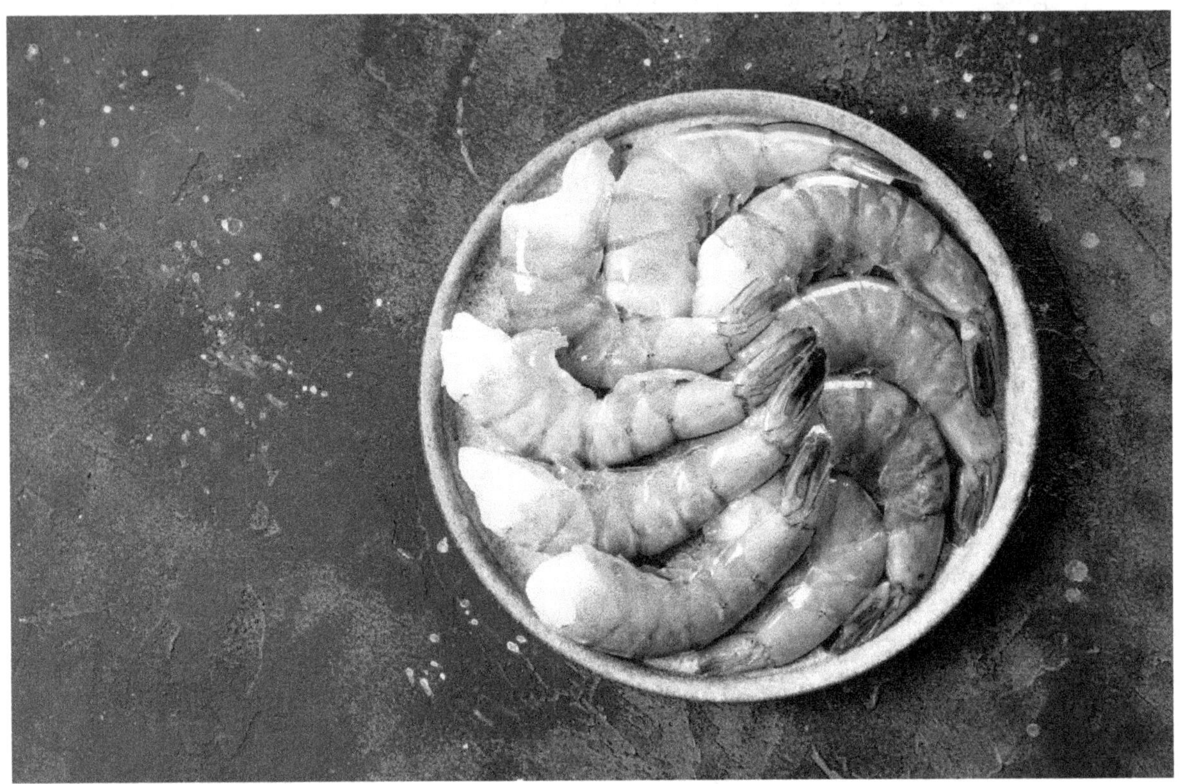

Seafood is the best food for healthy and good-looking skin. Shrimps are packed with natural minerals and essential nutrients, and they taste delicious too.

Duration: 20 minutes

Serving Size: 4

List of Ingredients:

- 16 to 20 large shrimps, deveined without a head but with a tail on
- ¼ cup of ghee, divided
- 2 tablespoons of minced garlic
- ½ teaspoon of minced ginger
- 1 red chili, finely chopped
- 1 teaspoon of black pepper or more for taste
- 2 large limes
- 1 cup of cilantro

AAAAAAAAAAAAAAAAAAAAA

Instruction:

A. Begin by preparing the creamy cilantro sauce. This sauce will add a flavorful and vibrant element to your dish.

B. In a pan, add half of the ghee and squeeze the fresh limes into it. This step infuses the ghee with tangy citrus flavors and creates a base for the sauce.

C. Gently bring the ghee and lime mixture to a simmer, allowing the flavors to meld together.

D. Add chopped cilantro to the pan and let it come to a boil for about 30 seconds to a minute. This quick cooking time helps retain the bright green color and fresh flavor of the cilantro.

E. Season the cilantro sauce with salt and pepper to taste. This adds the perfect balance of seasoning to enhance the overall taste of the sauce.

F. In the same pan, add the remaining ghee and sauté minced garlic, ginger, and chili. These aromatic ingredients contribute depth and warmth to the dish.

G. Introduce the shrimp to the pan and cook until they turn a delicate pink color. This indicates that the shrimp are cooked through and ready to be enjoyed.

H. Once the shrimp are cooked, transfer them to a serving bowl.

I. Drizzle the creamy cilantro sauce over the sautéed shrimp. The sauce will add a creamy, herby flavor to the dish, complementing the succulent shrimp.

J. Serve the Ghee Sautéed Shrimps with Creamy Cilantro Sauce as a flavorful and satisfying dish.

Cooking Notes:

- Making the cilantro sauce first ensures that you have a delicious accompaniment ready when the shrimps are cooked.
- Squeezing fresh lime into the ghee infuses the fat with citrusy tanginess that elevates the flavor of the dish.
- Adding cilantro to the ghee creates a vibrant green sauce with a fresh herbaceous taste.
- Boiling the cilantro briefly helps maintain its color and flavor without overcooking it.
- Adjust the amount of salt and pepper in the cilantro sauce according to your taste preferences.
- Sautéing garlic, ginger, and chili in ghee adds aromatic complexity to the dish.
- Cooking the shrimp until they turn pink indicates that they are fully cooked and tender.
- Drizzling the cilantro sauce over the cooked shrimp ensures that each bite is infused with flavor.
- This recipe combines rich flavors and textures for a delightful culinary experience.
- Always ensure that any ingredients used are safe and suitable for your intended audience's dietary preferences and restrictions.

- Detailed cooking notes help guide the preparation process and ensure a successful outcome.
- If you have dietary restrictions or preferences, you can customize the dish by using suitable substitutes or adjustments.
- Adjust spice levels according to personal preference, and consider the individual dietary needs and sensitivities of those you're serving.

25. Skin Bright Lemon & Lime Water

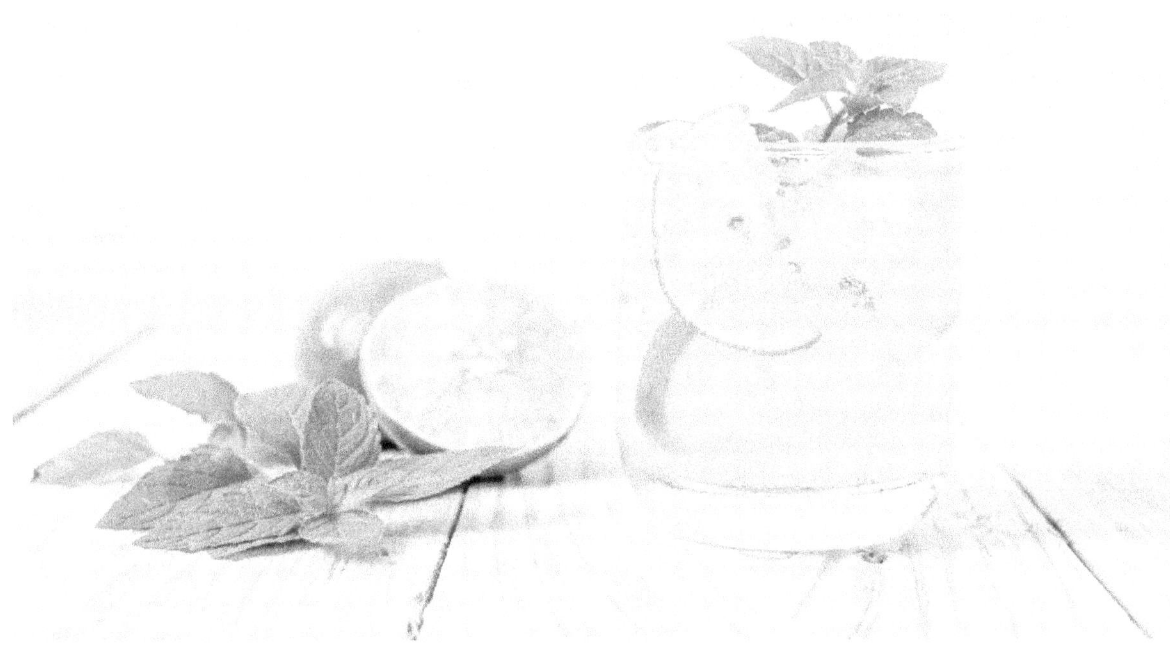

Lime and lemon's high Vitamin C content is the best way to maintain skin brightness and youthfulness. A glass every morning, warm or cold, is a good start to a wonderful day.

Duration: 5 minutes

Serving Size: 2

List of Ingredients:

- 1 medium-sized lemon
- 1 small lime
- 2 sprigs of mint
- 4 cups of sparkling water

AAAAAAAAAAAAAAAAAAAAAA

Instruction:

A. Begin by slicing the medium-sized lemon and the small lime. These citrus fruits will infuse your water with refreshing flavors.

B. Place the sliced lemon and lime into a jug. This jug will be the container for your skin-brightening lemon and lime water.

C. Pour the sparkling water over the sliced citruses in the jug. The sparkling water adds a fizzy and effervescent quality to the drink.

D. Add 2 sprigs of fresh mint leaves to the water. Mint leaves contribute a pleasant and aromatic element to the beverage.

E. Allow the ingredients to sit in the jug for about 2 to 5 minutes. During this time, the flavors from the citruses and mint leaves will meld with the sparkling water.

F. After the flavors have had a chance to infuse, your Skin Bright Lemon & Lime Water is ready to be served.

Cooking Notes:

- Slicing the lemon and lime is important for releasing their juices and flavors into the water.
- Choosing fresh and ripe citruses ensures that the water will have a vibrant and appealing taste.
- Using a jug to hold the ingredients allows for easy mixing and serving of the infused water.
- The sparkling water adds a bubbly and refreshing quality to the beverage. You can adjust the amount of sparkling water according to your preference for fizziness.
- Mint leaves contribute a fragrant and aromatic note to the drink. You can gently bruise the mint leaves before adding them to the water to release more of their flavor.
- Allowing the ingredients to sit in the jug for a few minutes lets the flavors infuse and develop, creating a more flavorful drink.
- You can customize the intensity of the citrus flavors by adjusting the quantity of lemon and lime slices.
- This Skin Bright Lemon & Lime Water is a hydrating and flavorful option, especially during warm weather or as a refreshing beverage.
- Make sure to use fresh, high-quality ingredients for the best taste and results.
- Feel free to experiment with other additions such as cucumber slices, berries, or even a touch of honey for added sweetness.
- Stay hydrated and enjoy the vibrant flavors of this infused water while benefiting from the natural properties of the citrus fruits.
- This recipe is a simple way to create a refreshing and visually appealing drink that can be enjoyed on various occasions.
- Consider personal preferences and dietary restrictions when making and serving infused waters.

26. Sweet and Spicy Pineapple-Chicken Skewers

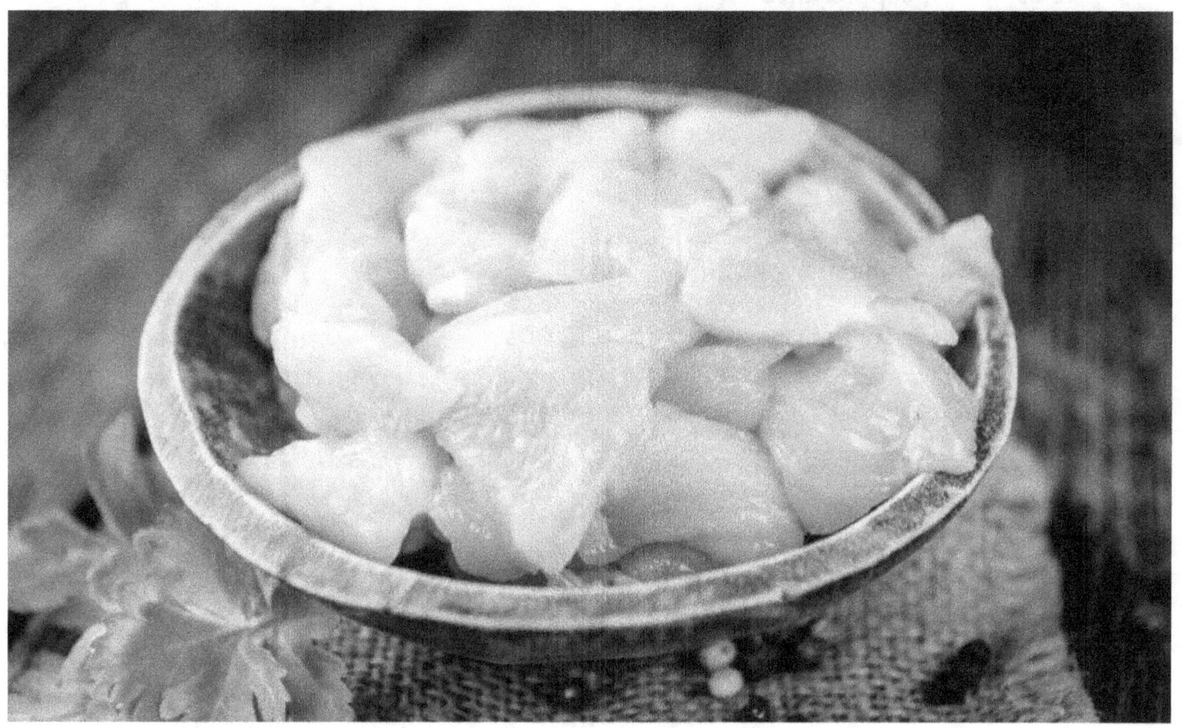

Pineapple is a sweeter way to increase collagen formation, and strengthen skin texture and elasticity without guilt.

Duration: 60 minutes

Serving Size: 4

List of Ingredients:

- 4 skinless chicken thighs boneless
- 1 teaspoon of garlic, minced
- 1 teaspoon of ginger, minced
- ½ cup of pineapple juice
- 1 teaspoon of chili flakes
- 1 small red, chili chopped
- 1 teaspoon of paprika
- 1 tablespoon of coconut oil
- 16 cubes of pineapple
- Sea salt

AAAAAAAAAAAAAAAAAAAAA

Instruction:

A. Begin by cutting each skinless, boneless chicken thigh into 4 pieces, resulting in a total of 16 pieces. This step ensures that the chicken is appropriately sized for skewering.

B. In a bowl, marinate the chicken pieces with the following List of Ingredients: minced garlic, minced ginger, pineapple juice, chili flakes, chopped red chili, paprika, and coconut oil. Make sure the chicken is coated well with the flavorful mixture. Allow the chicken to marinate for about 30 minutes, which enhances its taste and tenderness.

C. While the chicken is marinating, soak 4 skewers in water. Soaking the skewers prevents them from burning during the grilling process.

D. Once the chicken has marinated, it's time to assemble the skewers. Skewer 4 chicken pieces and 4 cubes of pineapple onto each soaked skewer. The combination of chicken and pineapple adds a delightful balance of flavors.

E. Preheat your grill before placing the skewers on it. This ensures that the skewers will be cooked evenly and thoroughly.

F. On the preheated grill, place the skewers and cook for approximately 5 minutes on each side. Keep an eye on the skewers to avoid overcooking or burning.

G. Once the chicken is cooked through and has a nicely grilled exterior, your Sweet and Spicy Pineapple-Chicken Skewers are ready to be served.

Cooking Notes:

- Cutting the chicken thighs into smaller pieces ensures that they cook evenly and are suitable for skewering.
- Marinating the chicken with the listed ingredients imparts flavor and tenderness. The pineapple juice adds a touch of sweetness and helps tenderize the meat.
- Soaking the skewers prevents them from catching fire or burning when placed on the grill.
- Assembling the skewers with alternating chicken pieces and pineapple cubes creates a visually appealing and flavorful combination.
- Preheating the grill is essential for achieving proper cooking and grill marks on the skewers.
- Cooking times may vary depending on the thickness of the chicken and the heat of the grill. Aim for juicy and fully cooked chicken without overcooking.
- Serve the skewers as a delicious appetizer, snack, or main dish. The sweet and spicy flavors are sure to be a hit.
- Adjust the level of spiciness by modifying the amount of chili flakes and chopped chili according to your preference.

- Ensure that the chicken is cooked to a safe internal temperature (165 degrees F or 74 degrees C) for consumption.
- Experiment with different marinade variations or additional ingredients like vegetables for a personalized touch.
- Grilling gives the skewers a smoky and charred flavor, but you can also cook them on a stovetop grill pan or in the oven if a grill is not available.
- Enjoy these Pineapple-Chicken Skewers as a delightful treat that combines the sweetness of pineapple with the savory flavors of marinated chicken.

27. Purple Blueberry Crumbly Cobbler

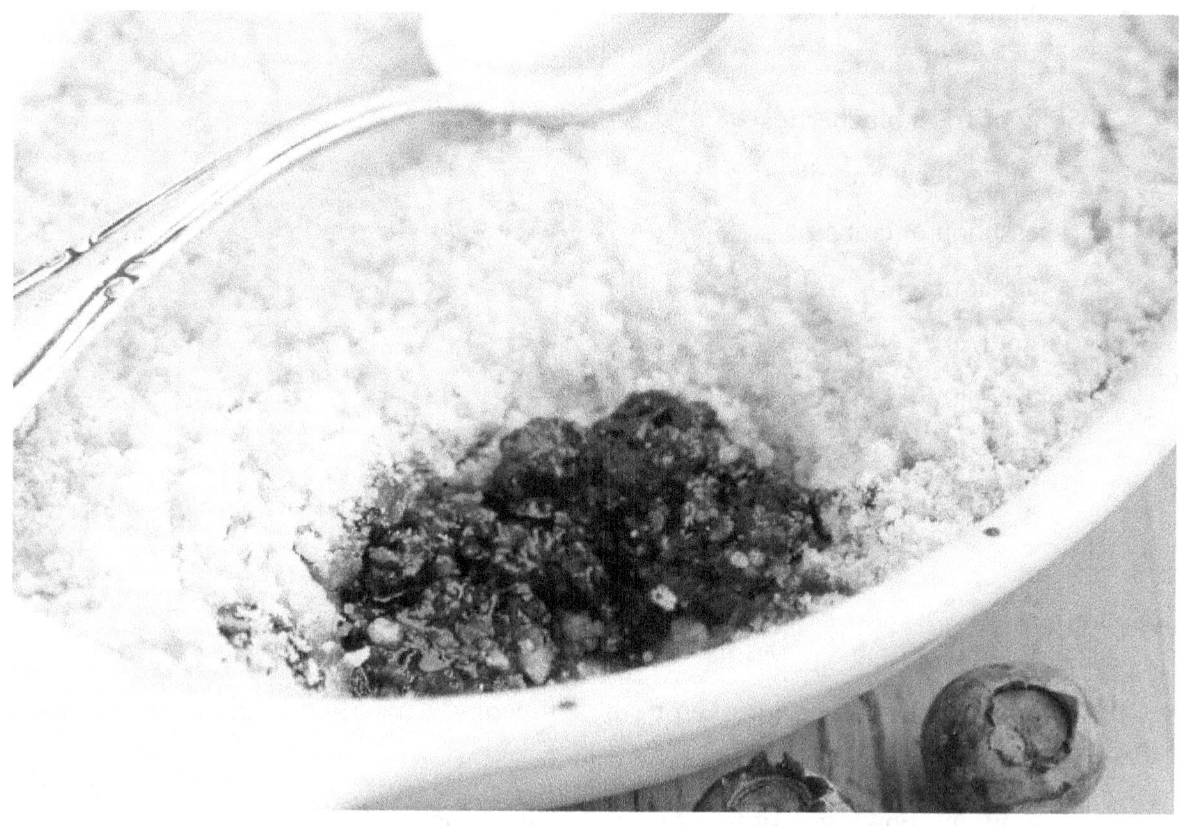

Kick stressed skin and wrinkles away with this delicious blueberry dessert, and it is super healthy too.

Duration: 35 minutes

Serving Size: 4 -6

List of Ingredients:

- ½ cup of rolled oats
- ½ cup of coconut flakes
- ¾ cup of oat flour
- 500g of fresh blueberries
- 1/3 cup of coconut oil
- ½ teaspoon of cinnamon
- ¼ cup of maple syrup
- 6 mint leaves chiffonade
- ¼ teaspoon of sea salt
- 1 sprig of rosemary

AAAAAAAAAAAAAAAAAAAAA

Instruction:

A. Begin by preheating your oven to the temperature specified in the recipe (usually around 350°F or 175°C).
B. In a mixing bowl, gently toss the fresh blueberries along with a handful of finely chopped fresh mint leaves. Transfer this fruity mixture into an oven-proof dish, ensuring an even distribution.
C. Introduce a fragrant element to the cobbler by placing a sprig of rosemary amidst the blueberries in the dish.
D. Now, it's time to prepare the crumbly topping. In another bowl, combine rolled oats, coconut flakes, oat flour, a drizzle of coconut oil, a pinch of aromatic cinnamon, a generous splash of maple syrup for sweetness, and a small amount of salt to enhance the flavors. Thoroughly mix these ingredients until they form a cohesive crumbly texture.

E. Gently spread the crumbly mixture over the blueberries in the oven-proof dish, creating an even layer that covers the entire surface.

F. Carefully place the dish into the preheated oven and allow the cobbler to bake for approximately 30 to 35 minutes. Keep an eye on it as it bakes, ensuring the topping turns golden brown and the blueberries release their juices, creating a bubbling filling.

G. Once the cobbler is baked to perfection, remove it from the oven and let it cool slightly before serving.

H. To serve, scoop out portions of the warm purple blueberry crumbly cobbler into dessert bowls. For an extra delightful touch, consider pairing each serving with a scoop of healthy coconut ice cream, which complements the flavors beautifully.

Cooking Notes:

- You can adjust the sweetness of the cobbler by modifying the amount of maple syrup according to your taste preferences.

- Feel free to experiment with other types of berries or fruits if you want to switch up the flavor profile.

- If you don't have oat flour, you can easily make your own by grinding rolled oats in a blender or food processor until they reach a fine consistency.

- Don't be afraid to get creative with the crumbly topping by adding chopped nuts, such as almonds or walnuts, for extra crunch and flavor.

- The rosemary sprig not only adds a lovely aroma but also a subtle earthy taste to the cobbler's filling. If you're not a fan of rosemary, you can omit it or replace it with a different herb.

- When serving, consider drizzling a touch of extra maple syrup on top for an added burst of sweetness and presentation appeal.

28. Dark Chocolate Silky Smooth Bites

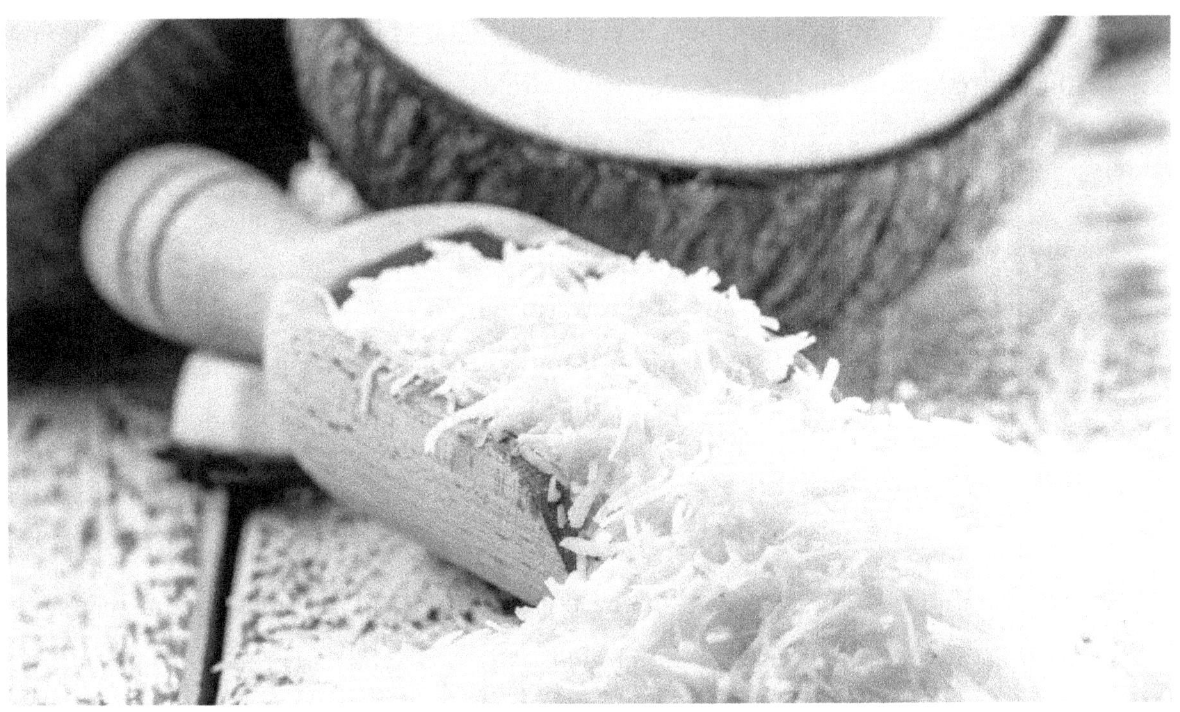

They may be bitter, but they lock in excellent properties to keep your skin supple by increasing blood flow to it.

Duration: 30 minutes

Serving Size: 12 – 16 bites

List of Ingredients:

- 2 ripe but firm bananas
- 1 cup of sweetened coconut flakes
- 1 ¼ cups of dark chocolate 70%
- ¼ cup of coconut oil
- Sea salt

AAAAAAAAAAAAAAAAAAAAAA

Instruction:

A. Begin by melting dark chocolate and coconut oil together. Stir the mixture until you achieve a velvety smooth texture that's free of any lumps or clumps.

B. Proceed to peel the bananas and cut them into rounds that are approximately ½ inch thick.

C. Place the banana rounds in a Ziploc bag along with the coconut flakes. Ensure the banana slices are thoroughly coated with the coconut flakes by gently shaking the bag.

D. Once the bananas are coated, transfer the Ziploc bag to the freezer and allow the banana slices to freeze. This step helps create a firm base for the chocolate coating.

E. Arrange the frozen banana slices on a rack or tray, preparing them for the next step.

F. For a convenient holding method, insert a toothpick into each frozen banana slice.

G. Take the toothpick-embedded banana slices and dip them one by one into the melted chocolate mixture. Make sure to coat each slice evenly with the smooth chocolate.

H. As the chocolate-dipped banana slices are lifted, give them a light sprinkle of sea salt, adding a delightful contrast of flavors.

I.   Once the chocolate-coated banana slices are ready, return them to the freezer for a second round of freezing. This helps solidify the chocolate coating and create a satisfying crunch when bitten into.

J.   Once fully frozen and the chocolate is firm, your dark chocolate silky smooth bites are ready to be enjoyed as a delectable treat.

Cooking Notes:

- Opt for high-quality dark chocolate for the best taste and texture in your silky smooth bites.
- When melting the chocolate and coconut oil, use a gentle heat method like a double boiler or microwave in short bursts, stirring frequently to prevent overheating.
- Ensure the banana slices are evenly coated with coconut flakes before freezing, as this adds an extra layer of texture and flavor.
- Using a toothpick to dip the banana slices makes the process cleaner and more manageable, and it provides a convenient handle for eating.
- The sea salt sprinkle adds a sophisticated touch by enhancing both the sweetness of the chocolate and the natural flavors of the banana.
- After the final freezing stage, transfer the silky smooth bites to an airtight container and store them in the freezer until you're ready to enjoy them.
- These bites are a wonderful way to satisfy a chocolate craving with a healthier twist, thanks to the natural sweetness of bananas and the indulgence of dark chocolate.

29. All the Good Stuff Stuffed Pepper

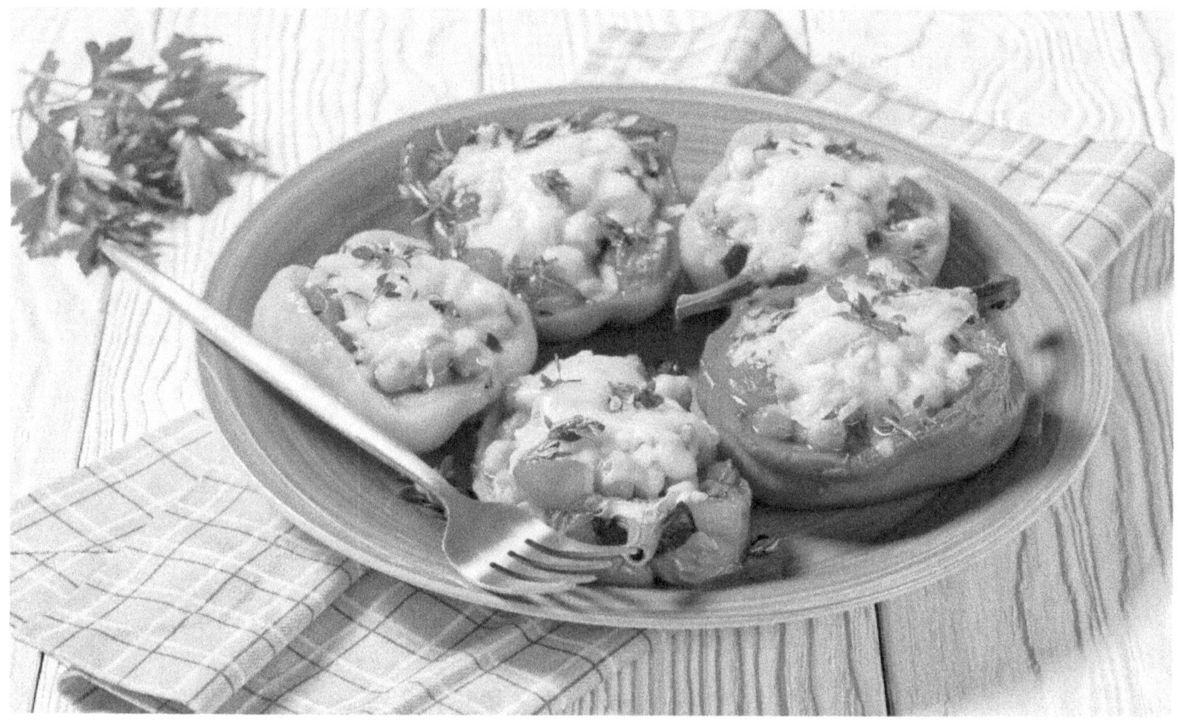

Peppers contain high vitamin C for collagen and power antioxidants too.

Duration: 30 minutes

Serving Size: 4

List of Ingredients:

- 1 cup of cooked brown rice
- 200g of ground beef
- 1 teaspoon of garlic minced
- 1 teaspoon of ginger minced
- 1 tablespoon of tomato paste
- 1 cup of chopped tomatoes
- 1 med-size red chili
- 1 small onion chopped
- 1 tablespoon of oil
- ½ a bunch of parsley
- 4 large bell peppers
- 1 large carrot cubed
- Salt and pepper

AAAAAAAAAAAAAAAAAAAAA

Instruction:

A. Begin by browning the beef in a non-stick pan until it's cooked through and has a rich color.

B. Add minced garlic, ginger, chopped chili, and diced onion to the pan. Sauté these aromatics until they become fragrant and the onion turns translucent.

C. Incorporate a drizzle of oil, tomato paste, chopped tomatoes, and diced carrot into the mixture. Stir everything together to combine the flavors.

D. Season the mixture with your choice of spices and let it cook for 2 to 5 minutes, allowing the ingredients to meld and develop depth of flavor.

E. Integrate the cooked rice into the pan, making sure to mix it well with the other ingredients. Then, gently fold in the freshly chopped parsley for a burst of freshness.

F. Proceed to stuff the prepared filling into the bell peppers, ensuring each pepper is generously filled with the flavorful mixture.

G. Place the stuffed peppers onto a baking tray, and cover them with foil to retain moisture and aid in even cooking. Bake the peppers in the preheated oven for about 20 minutes.

H. After the initial 20 minutes, remove the foil to allow the tops of the stuffed peppers to brown and develop a slight crispiness. Continue baking until the peppers are tender and the tops are golden.

I. Once cooked to perfection, carefully take the stuffed peppers out of the oven.

J. Serve the "All the Good Stuff" stuffed peppers as a hearty and wholesome meal that's filled with a delicious blend of flavors and textures.

Cooking Notes:

- Choose lean ground beef for a healthier option. You can also substitute ground turkey, chicken, or a plant-based protein if preferred.

- Adjust the amount of chili according to your heat preference. If you enjoy spicier food, you can add more chili or even include other hot peppers.

- When adding tomato paste, consider briefly cooking it with the aromatics to enhance its flavor before adding the chopped tomatoes.

- Feel free to customize the seasonings with herbs and spices that you enjoy. Common options include cumin, paprika, oregano, or thyme.

- Mixing the rice with the other ingredients ensures that the flavors are evenly distributed throughout the filling.

- Choose bell peppers that have a sturdy shape and can stand upright on the baking tray.
- The foil covering during the initial baking time helps steam the peppers and filling, ensuring they cook thoroughly and remain moist.
- Removing the foil for the final part of baking adds a desirable texture to the tops of the stuffed peppers.
- You can garnish the finished dish with additional chopped parsley or other fresh herbs for a burst of color and added freshness.
- These stuffed peppers can be served on their own as a complete meal or accompanied by a side salad for a well-rounded plate.

30. Summer Young Watermelon Salad

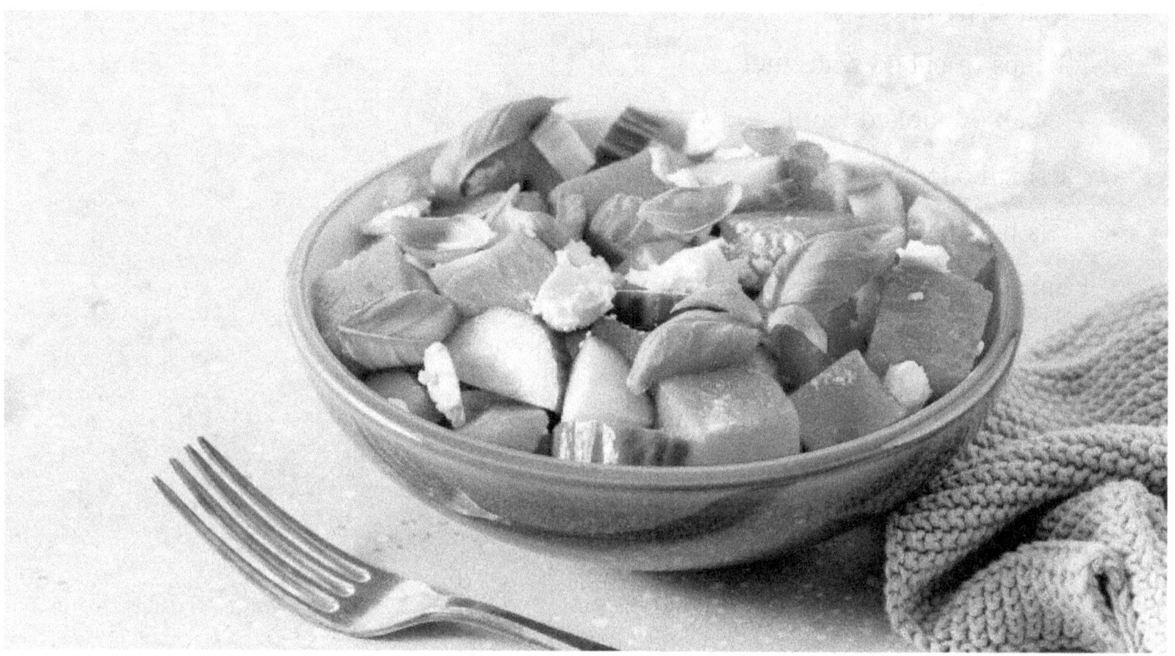

Lycopene is a great component that blocks UV rays from damaging the skin, and watermelon is a carrier of this magic substance.

Duration: 10 minutes

Serving Size: 2

List of Ingredients:

- 100g of baby broccoli stem
- 1 tablespoon of chopped walnuts
- 3 cups of cubed watermelon
- ½ cup of cooked lentil
- 1 small cucumber diced
- ½ a bunch of baby mint leaves
- Salt and pepper
- 150g of Feta cheese
- 1 tablespoon of olive oil
- 1 tablespoon of lemon juice

AAAAAAAAAAAAAAAAAAAAAA

Instruction:

A. Begin by steaming the broccoli in salted boiling water for a short period of 2 to 3 minutes. Once steamed, quickly cool the broccoli by immersing it in ice water. After cooling, gently pat the broccoli dry with a clean towel and proceed to chop it, including both the stems and florets.

B. In a bowl, combine the chopped broccoli with chunks of fresh watermelon and slices of cucumber. Add crumbled feta cheese and freshly torn mint leaves to the mix.

C. Season the salad with a pinch of salt and a sprinkle of black pepper, ensuring a balanced flavor throughout.

D. Introduce cooked and cooled lentils to the bowl, gently tossing all the ingredients together to evenly distribute the flavors and textures.

E. For the dressing, whisk together olive oil and freshly squeezed lemon juice until they are well combined. Drizzle this refreshing dressing over the assembled salad, adding a zesty and tangy element that ties the ingredients together.

F. Serve your vibrant and delightful summer young watermelon salad as a refreshing side dish or a light and healthy meal option.

Cooking Notes:

- Be careful not to overcook the broccoli during the steaming process. It should be tender yet still crisp. The ice water bath helps halt the cooking process and maintains the vibrant green color.
- When chopping the broccoli, consider cutting it into bite-sized pieces to ensure each forkful has a balanced mix of flavors and textures.
- Watermelon and cucumber provide a juicy and refreshing contrast to the other ingredients in the salad.
- Feta cheese adds a creamy and slightly tangy element that pairs well with the sweetness of watermelon and the earthiness of broccoli.
- Mint leaves bring a burst of freshness and aroma to the salad. Tear them rather than chop for better flavor release.
- The addition of lentils enhances the salad's nutritional value by providing protein and fiber. You can use cooked and cooled lentils from a can for convenience.
- The olive oil and lemon juice dressing not only adds a delightful flavor but also helps meld the ingredients together and enhances their natural tastes.
- Customize the dressing by adjusting the ratio of olive oil to lemon juice according to your preference for tanginess and richness.
- Consider adding toasted nuts or seeds, such as almonds or sunflower seeds, to introduce an extra crunch and a nutty flavor to the salad.
- This salad is versatile and can be enjoyed as a light lunch, a side dish for barbecues, or even as a potluck contribution for summer gatherings.

See You Again

Thank you for purchasing and reading my book. Your support means a lot, and I'm grateful you chose my book among many options. I write to help people like you, who appreciate every word.

Please share your thoughts on the book, as reader feedback helps me grow and improve. Your insights may even inspire others. Thanks again!